# HOW TO GET PREGNANT

# HOW TO GET PREGNANT

## Sherman J. Silber, M.D.

**WARNER BOOKS**

A Warner Communications Company

WARNER BOOKS EDITION

Copyright © 1980 by Sherman J. Silber
All rights reserved.

This Warner Books Edition is published by arrangement with
Charles Scribner's Sons, 597 Fifth Avenue, New York, N.Y. 10017

All the drawings in this book are by Scott T. Barrows

*Cover design by New Studio. Inc.*

Warner Books, Inc., 666 Fifth Avenue, New York, N.Y. 10103

A Warner Communications Company

Printed in the United States of America

First Warner Books Printing: November, 1981

10 9

**Library of Congress Cataloging in Publication Data**

Silber, Sherman J.
How to get pregnant.

Reprint. Originally published: New York:
Scribner, 1980.
Includes index.
1. Sterility. 2. Conception. I. Title.
RC889.S52 1981 616.6'92 81-2670
ISBN 0-446-38400-3 (USA) AACR2
ISBN 0-446-38401-1 (Canada)

# Contents

# Introduction

My six-year-old boy, David, recently explained to me his view of the facts of life. "First, you have to have a mommy and a daddy. The baby starts out as a little 'squirm' inside Daddy. Well, actually it's called a 'sperm.' It looks just like a tadpole. It swims through a tunnel in Mommy's belly. Then it finds her egg somehow and becomes a baby." Unfortunately, many adults don't understand this process much better than my little six-year-old. Yet 15 percent of American couples are infertile, and desperately desire to have children.

David then went on to ask, "Daddy, I don't really see how the sperm knows where to find the egg; and what if, when he gets there, there isn't any egg?" An answer to that seemingly simple question will help the majority of infertile couples to obtain their dream: a baby.

A couple's awareness of their inability to have children usually creeps up very slowly. A recent patient of mine had been on birth control pills for eight years, waiting until the day when she could plan to have a baby. When she finally discontinued the pill, the months and years went agonizingly by, with no pregnancy, and she cursed each menstrual period. Her husband was unwilling to have his sperm checked, because he felt that anyone as virile as he could not possibly be infertile. The patient herself had a routine gynecological examination which showed no abnormality, but the physician seeing her then had no particular interest in fertility. It was not until fifteen years after she had first started taking birth control pills (unnecessarily, after all) that she had an X ray which revealed blockage of her fallopian tubes—a problem which could have been corrected.

## Seeking Medical Advice

Although the infertile couple usually does well to seek prompt medical advice, the advice isn't always very good. I once had a patient who had been trying unsuccessfully to impregnate his wife for two years. His previous urologist was not particularly interested in infertility, considering it one of the annoying and abstruse segments of his practice. When the report came back from the lab showing a relatively low sperm count, with poor movement of the sperm, the doctor placed the patient on thyroid supplements—a therapy with no scientific basis, routinely used years ago. No attention was paid to a more likely factor, the varicose vein in his left testicle, which the doctor had not noticed.

When I first saw this patient, his sperm count was poor and his wife was still not pregnant. In fact, he had hyperirritability caused by an excess of the thyroid hormones he was taking. A very simple operative procedure involving tying off the varicose vein of his testicle resulted in a prompt increase in his sperm count to normal levels, and the movement of his sperm became vigorous. After discontinuing the thyroid pills, his irritability vanished. Three months later his wife became pregnant.

Correcting one partner's problem is not always the only answer. I recently saw a couple of whom the husband had had a similarly fruitless course of hormone therapy, neglecting the testicular varicose vein that was the major cause of his infertility. Furthermore, the wife had been told not to bother with tests, because of her husband's low sperm count. Nonetheless, I advised that the wife be examined by a gynecologist. It seemed unlikely that the gynecologist would turn up any problems, since her preliminary exam had been normal. Yet when he checked her with a laparoscope (a telescope used to examine a woman's internal sex organs) she was found to have a condition called endometriosis. When this was treated, she finally became pregnant.

## When to Have Intercourse

The problems of the infertile couple are not always this clinical, however. A knowledge of how the male makes and delivers his sperm, and how the female processes it, will make it clear to any couple that their patterns of intercourse and their timing of intercourse may be the only problem. I had one couple who were so anxious to have sex at just the "right time" that they went out and bought a basal body temperature thermometer to determine at exactly what time of the month the wife ovulated. With a very superficial understanding they then proceeded to withhold intercourse until after her temperature went up, indicating that she had ovulated. What they didn't realize is that for pregnancy to occur they should have had intercourse twenty-four hours earlier. Rather than maximizing their chances for pregnancy, ironically they were actually practicing rhythm birth control. It wasn't until they threw away their basal body temperature thermometer and had intercourse when they wanted it that pregnancy occurred.

On the other hand, it must be remembered that a woman is fertile only at a very precise interval of about forty-eight hours during any particular month. If the husband's sperm is not there in adequate quantity during that precise interval, then the entire month is wasted. If the husband is out of town on business on a regular basis during the midportion of her cycle, it is easy to see how years could pass by without any pregnancy, even though the couple has no true infertility problem.

## Ill-Considered Sterilization

Sometimes the infertility problem is self-induced by a premature or perhaps ill-considered sterilization procedure. Butch, for example, was a very hardworking but poor farmer who lived off the land in the northern California mountains. He built his own house, grew his own food, and had a beautiful outlook on life. He had two wonderful children, a boy and a girl, and though Butch and his wife had very little income, their life was ideal. They agreed that two children were enough, so Butch saved up enough money to go into town and have one of the local doctors perform a vasectomy on him. One month later his only son drowned. He was beside himself with grief. He knew that more children would not replace his tragically lost son, but still the world suddenly seemed to be coming apart.

Chuck had a somewhat different story. He and his wife knew all along that they would want only two children, since they wanted to provide the best in college education for both of them. They already had one child and the wife was eight months pregnant. Chuck figured that he ought to get a vasectomy before the delivery, so that his wife would not have to use any birth control measures afterward. They had no difficulty finding a surgeon who would perform this procedure. Then, one month later, the baby was stillborn.

Fortunately, these patients were able to have their vasectomies reversed by an intricate new microsurgical technique. Butch has a beautiful new baby boy, and though he and his wife have never forgotten their love for the child that was lost, their faith in the universe and their society has been restored. Chuck and his wife now have the second baby they always wanted. Luckily, both of these potentially tragic stories ended on a happy note.

Not every patient who has had a vasectomy even realizes that he has had one. Mike and Gordon, two patients of mine, both had hernias when they were infants. Twenty years ago, surgery on children was not nearly as refined as it is today, and when these tiny two-month-old babies were having their hernias repaired, neither they nor their well-meaning surgeons were aware of the fact that a relatively enormous segment of the vas deferens was accidentally being removed along with the hernia. In Mike's case, it wasn't until he was twenty-five years of age and found to be infertile that his inadvertent vasectomy was discovered. In Gordon's case, there had been two hernias, and the surgeon, who was his grandfather, died before he had a chance to operate on the second one. So Gordon luckily remained fertile on one side when he grew up.

## Understanding Your Reproductive Processes

Fortunately, the solution to most infertility problems is not so exotic or complicated. The couple must have an understanding of the whole process of reproduction if their fears are to be alleviated. Even for those who have no hope of pregnancy, at least a clear understanding of how their bodies work can prevent needless anxiety about whether or not they have gone far enough in their search. It is the goal of this book to explain in simple language with simple illustrations the roles of the man and the woman in achieving pregnancy. We'll discuss how the testicles work to make sperm, how the sperm reaches the ejaculate, and why hundreds of millions of sperm are necessary when it is only one single sperm that actually fertilizes the egg. Once the sperm have been deposited in the female, they have a long and arduous journey ahead of them, like salmon entering the mouth of a river to swim upstream to spawn. An equally incredibly complex series of events must take place in the female to prepare the egg for fertilization and then sustain it. These are events which anxious would-be parents need to comprehend. Every facet of your reproductive processes will be explained in this book in language you can understand and enjoy.

In addition, we will explore the outer limits of present fertility research. You will learn about the new experiments with artificial insemination, freezing and storage of sperm and embryos, test-tube babies, cloning, and the formation of a baby from the fusion of two eggs without any sperm at all.

It is not the goal of this book to teach couples in need of medical attention how to bypass that need and treat themselves. On the contrary, my goal in this book is to educate couples sufficiently so that they can find the appropriate physician and, as educated patients, aid in their own treatment. Many couples really are not infertile in a true sense and do not need medical attention. An understanding of how our bodies work may help such couples get through the brief interlude of doubt and concern that all of us go through when we do not achieve pregnancy the very first month we try.

With the liberalization of birth control measures and the legalization of abortions, very few unwanted babies are presently available for adoption in the United States. This has created an almost frantic concern that any child we get to rear will have to be our own. This anxiety in itself can often affect fertility. In the past, an infertile couple might adopt a child, and then, once their anxieties about becoming parents were relieved, the wife would get pregnant. Today, with so few babies available for adoption, the only way to relieve such anxiety is to acquire a solid understanding of fertility and infertility.

# ·1·

# The Female's Role

The journey which sperm must make through the female genitals to fertilize the egg, as well as the simultaneous adventure of the egg emerging from the ovary to be swallowed by the tube, fertilized, and then hustled along into the womb to implant, constitutes an incredible odyssey fraught with excitement and peril every step of the way. Failure of the sperm or egg to make an important connection anywhere along this complicated itinerary would spell sure death. Before we describe this terrifying journey, we will map out briefly in this section the structure of the female organs in which the adventure takes place.

## *The Vagina and Uterus*

The vagina is an elastic canal about four to five inches long, into which the male of course inserts his penis during intercourse. At the end of this canal is a structure called the cervix, where the entrance to the uterus, or womb, is located. When the doctor performs a pelvic exam by inserting the small metal instrument called a speculum, it is the cervix which he is observing in the deepest reaches of the vagina. The uterus is a hard, muscular, pear-shaped structure with a narrow triangular cavity inside, so small that it would barely hold a teaspoonful of fluid (Figs. 1 and 2). The cervix is the opening into the uterus. The fertilized egg implants itself in

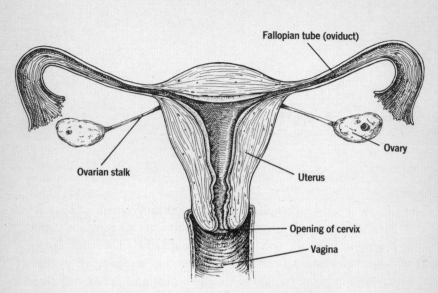

*Figure 1*. The Female Reproductive Organs.

the uterus and grows there during the next nine months into a full-term baby. The uterus has a remarkable capacity to expand in order to allow room for this growing baby. As it expands during the nine months of pregnancy, the uterus squashes and pushes aside all of the other organs of the abdomen. At the end of nine months, its muscles contract during labor to squeeze the baby out into the world.

## The Tubes and Ovaries

Far back in each corner of the uterus is a tiny canal that leads into the fallopian tube, or oviduct, the tube through which the egg must pass to reach the uterus. These little canals which connect the uterus with the tubes are only about one-seventieth to one-hundredth of an inch inside, about the diameter of a pinpoint. Each tube then widens into a large, flowerlike opening inside the

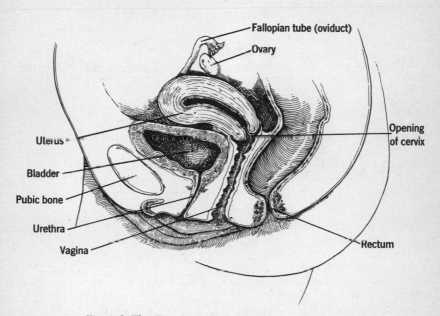

*Figure 2.* The Female Reproductive Organs (side view).

woman's body cavity. Both of the woman's tubes are about four inches long. The tubes hang freely in the abdomen and they are not connected directly with the ovaries (Fig. 3).

The ovaries are the organs which make the female's eggs and her major sex hormones. They sit outside the uterus and tubes, held by stalks called the ovarian ligaments. When an egg is extruded every month from the surface of one of the ovaries, it is released into the abdominal cavity rather than directly into the tube. The open end of the tube, called the fimbria, comes to life like an octopus tentacle when ovulation occurs, and actively grasps the egg after its volcanolike eruption from the ovary. The end of the tube thus actually reaches for the egg and swallows it, for transport ultimately to the womb.

Unlike the testicle, which is continually churning out billions of new sperm, the ovary never produces any new eggs. When a woman is born, she has within her ovaries all of the eggs that she

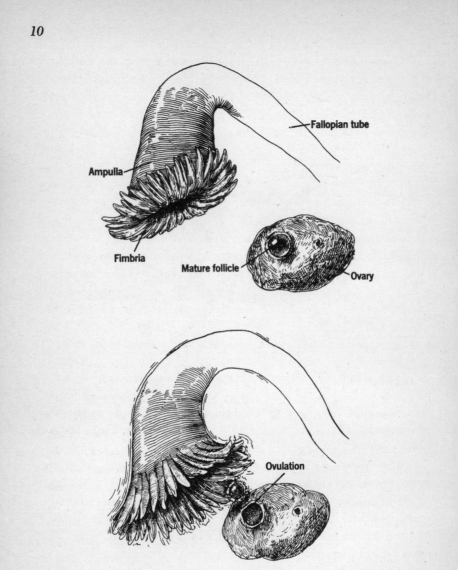

*Figure 3*. Ovulation.

will ever have. No new eggs are formed. While the male seems to wastefully produce billions of sperm every week from basic precursor cells called spermatogonia, the female simply matures one of her existing eggs for ovulation each month. She eventually runs out of this limited supply at the time of her menopause.

Ovulation is an event which takes place around the middle of the monthly cycle whereby an egg is extruded almost violently from the surface of an ovary into the abdomen. The eggs first must mature within an enlarging cavity in the ovary, called the follicle. The ovaries mature and release only about four hundred such eggs during the course of a woman's lifetime. When her stock of pre-made eggs is exhausted, her ovaries shrivel up, and she goes through what is called menopause, some time between the ages of forty-five and fifty-five. Generally, the most fertilizable eggs are released earlier in life. Thus with advancing years, though the woman may be fertile, her relative fertility diminishes.

The fact that the woman's eggs have already been manufactured and merely need to be properly extruded (whereas the male's sperm must be manufactured by a very temperamental assembly-line process) makes it much easier to treat fertility problems in the female than in the male. When a woman's clockwork goes wrong, and she ovulates improperly or not at all, it is usually not difficult to regulate her system with hormone or drug therapy. The eggs were already made decades before, and only require a little bit of guidance. However, in the male who is infertile because of insufficient sperm production, the situation is usually not as simple. For this reason, in many cases the husband's low sperm count is best handled by treatment of the wife in order to maximize her fertility potential. Hormonal manipulations to improve the woman's fertility are much more likely to be successful than hormonal manipulations of the man.

### How Does the Egg Reach the Tube?

The journey of the egg, or ovum, through the tube and finally into the uterus after fertilization is extraordinarily hazardous. The woman's tube is not simply a passive channel through which the egg is transferred. Many events must work in precise synchrony in order for successful pregnancy to occur.

The egg must first be picked up from the surface of the ovary at the time of ovulation and transported by the fimbria into the wide area of the tube called the ampulla. This portion of the tube then must transfer the egg rather rapidly to a narrow region called the isthmus. Fertilization takes place here, only halfway toward the womb, by sperm coming in from the uterus. Once fertilized, the egg must first be nourished for several days by the tube before it passes into the womb.

The fertilized egg, or embryo, cannot be allowed to pass into the womb until it is two or three days old. If the embryo is transferred into the uterus too soon, it will not be ready to implant, and it will die. If the transfer of the egg into the uterus is delayed too long, a "tubal," or "ectopic," pregnancy occurs (i.e., the fertilized egg implants in the tube rather than the womb). This eventually destroys the tube and requires surgery. Because the journey of the egg from the ovary to the site of fertilization, its nourishment in the tube, and the continuation of its journey into the womb are so intricate, problems with this transport process are frequently responsible for female infertility.

There are, on the surface of the fimbria, microscopic hairs called cilia, which constantly beat in a direction toward the uterus. The surgeon cannot really see these tiny little microscopic hairs no matter how closely he looks. Nonetheless, they are beating at a fantastically rapid speed and create a kind of conveyor-belt effect for moving the egg along the tube toward the uterus. When the egg is grasped by the fimbria, it is absolutely incredible to watch it being ushered along (almost like magic), disappearing into the tube. If you tried to pull the egg away from the fimbria as it slides rapidly into the tube, you would find that it requires a considerable amount of tug. It appears almost as though a mysterious force field is in operation, but actually it is the beating of these microscopic cilia that lure the egg into the tube within a matter of minutes.

The cilia dig into the sticky gel that surrounds the egg, called the cumulus oöphorus, and move the egg along by transporting the whole sticky, gooey mass, rather than by specifically moving the tiny egg. The egg itself is invisible to the naked eye, but the gel which surrounds it is easily visible. If this sticky substance were not present, and the egg were just placed bare upon the surface of the fimbria, the beating of the cilia would never move the egg along. The cilia are only able to dig in and transport the egg if there is this sticky, gooey material encasing it.

Because the ovary hangs freely in the abdominal cavity, it would seem remarkable that the egg ever gets into the tube. You would think that the egg would just fall off the ovary and be lost. However, the diligently maneuvering fimbria, like tentacles at the end of the tube, sweeps over the surface of the ovary at the time of ovulation and literally swallows the egg. The numerous cilia on the surface of the fimbria beat at a rate of twelve hundred times per minute and account for the fimbria's incredible grasping power.

The process of grasping the egg and moving it into the interior of the tube requires only about fifteen to twenty seconds. Once the egg is safely within the tube, it is transported within five minutes to the narrow region located halfway toward the uterus. Here, the egg must sit and wait for a successful sperm to challenge his way into her outer membrane, making a direct hit and thereby establishing pregnancy. While the egg is held in this position by the tight resistance of the narrow region of the tube, sperm are nonetheless able to travel in the opposite direction from the uterus.

The fertilized egg is then retained in the tube for several days while it goes through the very earliest stages of development. Once the egg has been allowed to develop in the tube for about two days, it passes rather rapidly into the uterus.

After the egg is released from the ovary, it is only "fresh," and thus capable of fertilization, for six to eight hours. If the egg is not penetrated by sperm soon after ovulation, it becomes overripe and dies. The likelihood of intercourse taking place during a specific eight-hour interval during any month is rather slight. So nature must provide some mechanism for providing a continuous flow of healthy sperm into the site of fertilization. That way, if intercourse is perhaps one or two days off the eight-hour limit, some sperm can still arrive at the site of fertilization at the right time.

For this reason, seemingly complicated barriers to sperm transport are necessary, not just as a senseless obstacle course designed to confound anxious parents-to-be. Rather, there must be a steady, continuous flow of a small number of sperm into the site of fertilization instead of a sudden, brief flooding with sperm before the egg is available. The success of test-tube fertilization demonstrates that, if eggs can be recovered at precisely the right time, they can be fertilized in the laboratory with only a small number of sperm. Then the complicated mechanism provided by nature to allow a slow, continuing flow of a small number of sperm at a time is not necessary, and the large numbers of sperm normally required for fertilization through intercourse are not needed.

## How Do Sperm Reach the Egg?

### EJACULATION INTO THE VAGINA

Most of the spermatozoa in the ejaculate are contained in the first portion which squirts out of the penis and enters the vagina. Thus at the moment of ejaculation the female's cervix, the opening leading into her womb, is bathed by a high concentration of sperm. Sperm begin to invade the very thick fluid called cervical mucus, which protects this opening to the womb, within just a few minutes after ejaculation (Fig. 4). The sperm must be able to invade the cervix by virtue of their own swimming ability. Nothing about the sexual act will help those sperm get into the cervix. They simply have to swim in on their own, and this requires a great deal of coordinated, cooperative activity on their part.

Ejaculation is a very tense moment for the sperm, as the vagina presents a very harsh, acid environment which would normally immobilize them quickly. The alkalinity of the semen (the fluid which contains the sperm), as well as the alkalinity of the cervical mucus, allows the sperm to survive in this difficult vaginal environment. However, even the semen is a potentially dangerous milieu for the sperm; although the semen confers an instant burst of activity to the sperm, any sperm that remain in semen for over two hours are likely to deteriorate. In order to survive long enough to

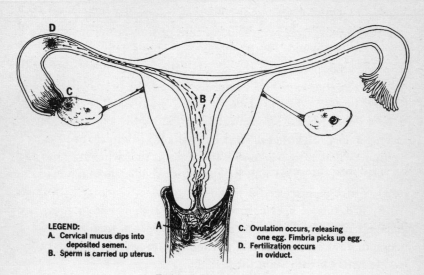

LEGEND:
A. Cervical mucus dips into deposited semen.
B. Sperm is carried up uterus.
C. Ovulation occurs, releasing one egg. Fimbria picks up egg.
D. Fertilization occurs in oviduct.

*Figure 4.* Fertilization.

get to the egg and fertilize it, the sperm must gain rapid access to the cervical mucus. Any sperm that have not penetrated the cervical mucus within one half hour after orgasm will not be able to do so later on, because by then they will have lost their ability to swim into the more friendly environment of the cervix. The invasion must take place promptly, and any sperm left behind will never be able to catch up.

### INVASION OF THE CERVICAL MUCUS

When the semen is deposited in the vagina, the first barrier which must be overcome is the cervix. In a sense even the vagina, though receptive to the penis, can be considered a barrier. Unless the sperm are deposited directly over the cervix, they face hostile vaginal secretions which can easily kill them. The deposition of semen in close proximity to the cervix thus undoubtedly aids the sperm in their rapid invasion of the cervix. Spermatozoa can be seen invading the cervical mucus within seconds after ejaculation. But most will not make it. Of some 200 million sperm deposited into the vagina near the cervix, only one-tenth of a million ever get into the womb. Thus over 99.9 percent of the sperm never have a chance of getting beyond the vagina.

Once the sperm enter the canal of the cervix, they are capable of fertilizing the egg for as long as forty-eight hours. They may actually live for up to six days, but they seem capable of fertilization for only two days after intercourse. Since the egg is only fertilizable for six to eight hours after ovulation, it is important to have a continuing flow of sperm across the tube so that whenever the egg reaches the area, there will be sperm available. In this sense the canal of the cervix can be looked upon as a receptacle through which platoons of spermatozoa migrate and in which some are detained in order to ensure a continuous supply of smaller numbers, over a more prolonged period of time, to the deeper recesses of the female where fertilization takes place.

Of course, these delaying mechanisms can occasionally do more harm than good in infertile couples if events do not allow the invasion of sperm to be mounted successfully. To understand how this invasion of sperm gets launched effectively, we must first understand that remarkable liquid which covers the opening of the womb, the cervical mucus. The cervical mucus presents a very effective barrier to bacteria and thus protects the womb against infection. It is a selective filter which favors normally active sperm, and excludes other objects (including poor-quality sperm) from access. It doesn't even permit access to normal sperm except during a specific period at mid-cycle, when ovulation is imminent and fertilization is possible. Cervical mucus resembles a thick, clear liquid which could be poured (like any liquid) from one container into another. However, in a technical sense it is not a liquid. As it is being poured, it can actually be cut with a scissors, just like a strand of plastic. In fact, if one wished to pour only a portion of the cervical mucus from one tube into another, it would be impossible without literally cutting it with a scissors. Thus, although it seems to behave as a thick liquid, it also has the characteristics of a very pliable, transparent plastic.

The amount of cervical mucus is very scanty just before and

just after menstruation. Within four days after the menstrual period has ceased, the cervical mucus gradually becomes more abundant until around the middle of the cycle, when ovulation is about to occur. At this time about ten times as much cervical mucus is pouring out of the opening of the womb as one would see either at the beginning or the end of the monthly cycle. In addition, cervical mucus becomes almost optically clear at this time, although it is translucent at other times. At the moment when fertilization is possible, near the time of ovulation, the cervical mucus can be stretched out into a very thin strand without breaking, but at other times in the cycle it is more sticky, and instead of stretching, it will break. All these changes in the cervical mucus which occur around the mid-cycle are designed to help sperm gain access to the womb. The more liquidlike character, the greater transparency, and the greater stretchability (called *spinnbarkheit)* are all characteristics which favor the successful invasion of an army of sperm. When the mucus is sticky and thick, not so abundant, and translucent rather than transparent, it is difficult if not impossible for any sperm to gain access.

Microscopically, the cervical mucus consists of a dense mesh of invisible fibrils which during most of the monthly cycle intertwine in a network that represents a solid barrier to invasion. Just prior to ovulation, under the effect of the female hormone estrogen, the amount of mucus production rises tenfold and the water content of the mucus increases. The otherwise dense and impenetrable microscopic fibrillar mesh gives way to a more open microscopic structure with much larger gaps between the fibrils. The molecules of the mucus then become arranged in parallel rows longitudinally along the canal of the cervix. The parallel arrangement encourages the sperm to move in one direction rather than in a haphazard motion. This is critical for a successful invasion of sperm.

When the semen reaches the cervical mucus just after ejaculation, a clear line can be seen separating the two different fluids. Soon, however, "phalanges" of sperm begin to penetrate this mucus, forming branching structures which invade deeply into it. Observing the sperm's attack on the cervical mucus under the microscope is an exciting event. Sperm at first seem to bounce against the cervical mucus without any evidence that they will ever be able to gain access. Furthermore, their movements while in the ejaculate are haphazard, not specifically aimed toward the mucus. However, within a matter of minutes one or two spermatozoa in a given area can be seen to make an indentation in the line separating the cervical mucus from the ejaculate. Once one sperm has been able to initiate the penetration of the mucus, other sperm quickly follow at exactly that point of entry. The sperm then continue to invade the cervical mucus much like a single-file line of army ants. Only one or two spermatozoa can pass at a time through this line of entrance.

Once initial penetration has occurred, more sperm are able to continue easily across this beachhead into the cervix. They swim in a straightforward direction along the parallel row of cells representing the microscopic molecular structure of the mucus. Once into the mucus, sperm are directed forward by the molecular structure of this remarkable liquid. Sperm which can only move in a curved path, or wiggle in place, are incapable of taking part in this invasion of the cervix, and are always left behind in the vagina to die.

Once this beachhead has been established, sperm swim through the cervical mucus at a speed of about one-eighth of an inch per minute. Thus, in about thirty minutes sperm can travel almost four inches, which is the distance required to reach the fallopian tubes. Even though only one of the two fallopian tubes will contain an egg during each cycle, the sperm enter both tubes. However, pregnancy would not be likely if all the sperm got into the fallopian tubes at one time, because they would soon pass on into the abdominal cavity. Unless they were lucky enough to pass through the fallopian tube at exactly the moment of ovulation, or within six to eight hours of that time, they would be long gone by the time the egg arrived. Thus nature had to invent some mechanism for allowing a continuous assault upon the site of fertilization by a smaller number of sperm.

Some of the sperm are transported rapidly and directly into

the uterus, but most of the sperm are led into "crypts," or little cavities, along the inside wall of the cervix, where they are stored. There is then a slow release of the spermatozoa from these storage sites. Thus the cervix acts as a reservoir from which, over a period of time, spermatozoa are slowly released into the uterus.

## TRAVELS OF THE SPERM THROUGH THE UTERUS

Scientists are not entirely sure whether sperm reach the fallopian tube purely on the basis of their own swimming motion or whether they are aided by contractions of the uterus, possibly induced by the woman's orgasm. These contractions do not seem to be absolutely necessary, because sperm deposited without intercourse in the cervical canal are quite capable of reaching the site of fertilization.

Once sperm reach the opening to the tube, they are detained again, and only slowly allowed to enter in relatively small numbers. In fact, only about four hundred out of the two hundred million sperm that started the attack ever get beyond this point. This gateway from the uterus into the tube appears to act as a dam, slowly releasing sperm into the oviduct over a period of time, and thus ensuring that some sperm are continually present at the site of fertilization. Since the cilia of the oviduct are rapidly beating in the direction of the uterus, the sperm that get past this entrance must swim upstream against the current in order to reach the egg.

## CAPACITATION OF SPERM

During the course of their odyssey toward the site of fertilization, the sperm undergo a process called capacitation, which is not fully understood. In fact, quite frankly, it is a mystery. Unless sperm reside for a certain period of time outside the male reproductive tract, for some unknown reason they are not capable of fertilization even though in every other respect they look normal. It used to be thought that this process of capacitation could only occur in the specific fluids of the female reproductive tract while the sperm migrate on their journey toward the egg. However, the recent scientific work with test-tube fertilization has demonstrated that capacitation of sperm (until now considered one of the greatest problems in successfully achieving test-tube babies) can occur in relatively simple fluids available in any laboratory. Thus the sperm seem to have a natural tendency toward developing their own capacitation for fertilization, and this simply requires a period of several hours. The old concept that this can only happen to sperm while they are journeying through the female tract has to be discarded. The fact that sperm require time to be capacitated could represent still another reason for the delaying mechanisms which the sperm encounter before gaining entrance into the tube where fertilization of the egg finally takes place.

### Ovulation

All of the eggs a woman ever releases were actually made years earlier, while she was still in her mother's womb. In men, sperm production continues every day by the millions, but a woman starts her life with only about 400,000 eggs, and that is all she will ever have. After she reaches the age of menstruation, each month one of her eggs develops sufficient maturity to be released and offered to the tubes for fertilization. Only about four hundred such eggs will be released during her lifetime. During each of these menstrual months, for every egg which is successfully developed and extruded, there are about one thousand that try to develop but instead lose the race and die. Thus, each month from one thousand eggs one is selected that will mature to the point where it can be extruded and fertilized. Each month, the ovulated egg may come from either of the two ovaries; it is a matter of chance which ovary will successfully mature a follicle during a given cycle. Somewhere between ages forty-five and fifty-five, she will run out of these eggs, and go through the menopause.

The process whereby a matured egg is extruded from the ovary is called ovulation. Since the majority of women who seem unable to have children owe their problems to a disturbance in ovulation, we should understand how this repeatable, monthly series of changes takes place in the ovary. Then later we will unravel the hormonal events which regulate the clocklike orderliness of the menstrual cycle. All of the events taking place during the month between menstrual periods are directed at preparing the womb and the cervix for the moment of ovulation, so that the sperm and the egg have the best opportunity for joining up and resulting in a baby.

FORMATION OF THE FOLLICLE

From the time of sexual maturity on, about one thousand undeveloped eggs, or oocytes, each month leave their prolonged resting phase and start to mature. This initiation of development is a continuous process, in marked contrast to ovulation, which occurs only once a month. Once the egg starts to develop, it proceeds inexorably, and no longer has the choice of returning to being quiescent. It either wins the race to ovulate, or it must degenerate and die.

The most striking feature of the egg's development is the growth of its surrounding compartment, called the follicle (Fig. 5). The growth of this follicle is stimulated by the hormone FSH (follicle-stimulating hormone) produced by the pituitary gland in the early phases of the monthly cycle. The time required for the egg to develop the proper follicle necessary for ovulation is about fourteen days. Although the follicle-stimulating hormone stimulates all of the developing eggs during the month to form follicles, one of the eggs always gets a head start over the others, and once it obtains that lead it never relinquishes it. The other eggs developing that month then degenerate.

The follicle is a spherical, bubblelike structure which bulges up from the surface of the ovary, and which contains the egg within a mass of sticky fluid. Occasionally two follicles successfully reach maturity, and they are both ovulated. In that circumstance the woman may have fraternal, or nonidentical, twins. Indeed, some of

22

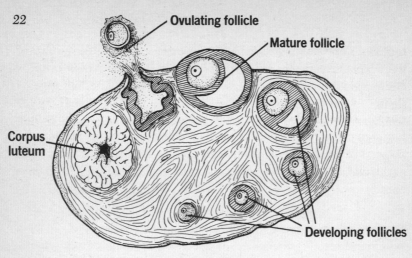

*Figure 5.* The Ovary.

Corpus luteum

Ovulating follicle

Mature follicle

Developing follicles

the drugs used to stimulate ovulation in women who would not otherwise ovulate may work better than expected, and cause the development of more than one follicle. Therefore, multiple births are somewhat more common in women who require medical treatment to help them ovulate.

Two or three days prior to mid-cycle, when the follicle has reached its maximum size, it produces an enormous amount of estrogen. This huge, dramatic increase in estrogen production stimulates the pituitary glands to release another hormone, LH (luteinizing hormone). This sudden release of LH is what triggers ovulation.

In this one respect the female brain is quite different from that of the male. In the female brain, the increase in estrogen causes the release of a hormone which triggers ovulation. In the male brain, an increase in estrogen would stop the release of this hormone. If an ovary were transplanted into a male it would never ovulate because the male's brain would not allow it.

RELEASE OF THE EGG

Under the influence of the mid-cycle LH surge, the wall of the follicle weakens and deteriorates, and a specific site on its surface ruptures. The bulging follicle is then extruded from the surface of the ovary through this ruptured area (Fig. 5). The whole event is quite dramatic. Observed under a microscope, ovulation appears similar to the eruption of a volcano. Occasionally women actually feel several hours of discomfort in their lower abdomen during ovulation. This discomfort is called *mittelschmerz*. In women who require hormone treatment to stimulate ovulation, the follicle may sometimes grow so large that when ovulation occurs it is extremely violent, and they may even become sick enough on occasion to require several days of rest in the hospital. We will discuss this in more detail in the chapter on treatment of the female. To ease your mind for the moment, however, this sort of complication is not very likely with modern dosage monitoring. It is mentioned only to underscore what a dramatic intra-abdominal event ovulation is.

PRODUCTION OF PROGESTERONE

The ruptured, empty follicle then undergoes another dramatic change, called luteinization. Prior to ovulation, the follicle had produced only estrogen. After ovulation, it produces the other female hormone, progesterone. Before ovulation occurred, it was impossible for the follicle to make progesterone. The production of progesterone forms the basis for all our methods of evaluating ovulation.

The rupture of the follicle at ovulation transforms it into a completely different endocrine gland, which manufactures a different female hormone and has an entirely different purpose. The new endocrine organ that forms from the ruptured follicle is called the corpus luteum. This is Latin for "yellow body" and simply signifies that the follicle turns yellow as it changes its identity. As soon as the corpus luteum begins to produce progesterone, the cervical mucus (which had become maximally receptive to sperm invasion just prior to ovulation) suddenly becomes sticky and totally impermeable to the invasion of sperm. In addition, progesterone causes the entrance of the cervix to close dramatically, even though just prior to ovulation it had been gaping in readiness for the entry of sperm.

Although estrogen stimulates the buildup of a thick, hard layer of endometrium to line the uterus prior to ovulation, this lining would not be receptive to the fertilized egg unless progesterone first had an opportunity to soften it. The corpus luteum manufactures this progesterone over a very limited time, however. If no pregnancy develops, the corpus luteum ceases to produce progesterone by ten to fourteen days after ovulation. With this cessation of hormone output by the ovary, the soft lining, which was built up in the womb to prepare for the nourishment of the baby, is shed and the woman menstruates. Then, with the development of a new follicle stimulated by a new increase in FSH, estrogen production resumes, and the cycle begins again.

The presence of progesterone only implies that ovulation has probably occurred. What this actually means is that a follicle has been ruptured and a corpus luteum has been formed. Ovulation may not have taken place. The hormone LH may stimulate the transformation of a follicle into a corpus luteum even though a proper egg may not have been released or picked up by the fallopian tube. All of the methods we have for determining whether or not a woman has ovulated (and indeed for pinpointing the time of her ovulation) are indirect, and based solely on the assumption that when progesterone is produced by the ovary, ovulation must have occurred. However, we have no direct clinical way of telling whether a woman has truly ovulated. We can only tell this indirectly by the presence of progesterone. That is why if the sequence of events in a woman's cycle indicates any delay in the production of progesterone, we must be suspicious of whether ovulation has truly occurred, or, if it has occurred, of whether the quality of the egg was adequate for fertilization.

# The Menstrual Periods—What Do They Mean?

SEX AND THE MONTHLY CYCLE

There are only one or two days in any given month when the female is very fertile; that is, when intercourse has a good chance of leading to pregnancy. This fertile period occurs just prior to ovulation. One of the most effective ways of making pregnancy more likely is to have intercourse take place around this fertile period of the month. In comparing humans to the rest of the animal kingdom, there is nothing unusual about the female's being fertile only during a limited period of the month. What should be surprising is that we are the only animal that enjoys sex continuously throughout the month without any regard to whether it is likely to lead to a baby. The female of most species will accept a male only for a very brief period, around the time of ovulation, when conception is most probable. This is called behavioral estrus, or heat. When the female is not in heat, she is completely uninterested in sex, or even actively hostile toward any male that approaches her.

In the wild, the females of many species become sexually receptive only once a year, and if they fail to conceive at that proper moment in the year, sexual receptivity does not occur again until the next breeding season. In other animals, receptive cycles of heat may recur at several intervals within a single breeding season, or continue monthly throughout the year. The structure and activity of the female tract in all animals changes cyclically in order to allow maturation of the egg, and preparation of the womb for reception of the fertilized egg.

The cycles which animals go through are called estrus cycles. No animals except for man and the apes have menstrual cycles. In a menstrual cycle the buildup of the lining of the womb is so lush, and the drop in hormone level supporting that lining is so abrupt, that at the end of the cycle the lining actually sheds and the woman bleeds for four to five days in what is commonly known as her "period." In all other animals, however, this shedding does not occur, and the lush lining of the womb merely returns to the thinned-out condition which marks the beginning of the next cycle. Even monkeys (who, like humans, menstruate, and who appear to have a reproductive pattern similar to humans') have a specific time in the cycle just prior to ovulation when the female is most interested in sex.

But in all animals except for humans there is no interest in sex until the time of heat, which is just prior to ovulation. Thus animals do not have to worry about when they ovulate in order to increase the likelihood of pregnancy. Nature has taken care of their timing for them. There are a few animals that are slightly different, in that the female is almost always receptive (such as the rabbit and the cat). However, in these cases the act of intercourse actually induces ovulation. Rabbits and cats will not ovulate except in response to the sexual act. So even the occasional rabbit with fertility problems need not worry about the timing of intercourse. In fact, "rhythm" birth control could never work with her. In all animals except man, sex appears to have just one purpose, and only occurs when that purpose is likely to be fulfilled.

Therefore, the concept of sex as a truly pleasurable event which may occur at any time is uniquely human. At the same time, however, human beings uniquely find it very difficult to know, without benefit of special tests, when they have ovulated or when intercourse is most likely to lead to pregnancy.

A number of biologists speculate that one of the distinguishing features of human life is the enduring family unit which facilitates the transmission of learning over hundreds of generations. One reason our civilization has achieved ascendancy over other animals is the continuity of learning provided by this stable family unit. Conceivably the continual enjoyment of sex, unrelated to heat and the necessity for reproduction, is one factor that has held our family units so closely together. This theory is pure speculation; but it emphasizes that we should not be disturbed by the difficulty of knowing when to have intercourse in order to get pregnant, but rather should be happy that an inclination toward intercourse does not specifically depend on the relatively infrequent event of ovulation.

HORMONES AND MENSTRUATION

Since most women are unaware of when they ovulate, we must try to understand the events in the menstrual cycle more fully than do our animal friends, who simply "do it" at the right time automatically. We will arbitrarily call the first day of the menstrual cycle "day one." Day one is the day that bleeding commences. Menstruation normally takes place over about four to five days. Thus the fourth day of bleeding would be the fourth day of the menstrual cycle. Bleeding usually ceases by day four or five and in most cases resumes about twenty-three to twenty-five days later, namely on day twenty-eight to day thirty of the cycle. Although the first day of menstruation represents a shedding of the lining of the womb that has built up in the previous month's cycle, it is actually the beginning of the next cycle.

On the first day of menstruation the hormone FSH is already stimulating development of a follicle that will take precedence over all other follicles trying to get started for the next month (see the chart "Hormone Changes Associated with Normal Ovulation"). FSH, which in females causes the follicle to develop, is the exact same hormone which in males helps to stimulate sperm production. As the follicle develops over the next ten to fourteen days, it produces increasing amounts of the female hormone estrogen, but no progesterone. The estrogen in turn slows down pituitary production of FSH, so that the FSH level begins to drop prior to ovulation. By day twelve to day fourteen of the menstrual cycle, the follicle is usually quite ripe and appears on the surface of the ovary as a fluid-filled bubble ready to burst. In the meantime the estrogen which has been produced by the follicle during this first half of the cycle is stimulating the uterus to prepare a lush lining to receive the fertilized egg. This first half of the cycle is called "proliferative." The estrogen has also caused the cervix to produce enormous quantities of optically clear mucus, with high water content, maximum elasticity, and the greatest receptivity to sperm penetration. Furthermore, the entrance to the cervix, which is generally closed, has begun to open between day nine and day four-

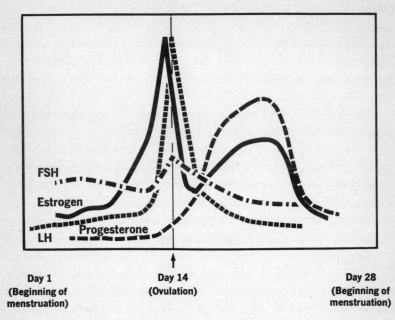

FSH

Estrogen

Progesterone

LH

Day 1
(Beginning of
menstruation)

Day 14
(Ovulation)

Day 28
(Beginning of
menstruation)

Hormone Changes Associated with Normal Ovulation.

teen, to the point where it is almost gaping with an abundant outflow of clear mucus just prior to ovulation. Estrogen has prepared the way.

The final effect of estrogen (in high quantities) is to trigger the release of a hormone from the primitive area of the brain, the hypothalamus, which causes the pituitary to release LH. This enormous release of LH then causes the follicle to burst, and ovulation occurs.

After ovulation the ruptured follicle forms the yellow corpus luteum which produces progesterone, the hormone of pregnancy. Over the next ten to fourteen days progesterone makes the lining of the uterus delicate and spongy, so that it can adequately nourish the fertilized egg. This second half of the cycle is called the "secretory" phase and is under the domination of progesterone. It is sometimes also called the "luteal" phase because progesterone is produced by the corpus luteum. If the egg is not fertilized, the corpus luteum has a very specific limited lifetime of ten to fourteen days. At the end of that time, if the woman is not pregnant the ovary stops producing progesterone, and the uterine lining can no longer support itself and sheds on what becomes day one of the next cycle.

As we shall see later, women can have all the machinery necessary to produce the right hormones and a proper egg, and yet not be fertile simply because the precise synchrony of events required to regulate the system is misfiring. It is as if a fine automobile were missing its spark plugs and points. The role of hormonal therapy in women with this problem is not to replace a deficiency in hormone production, but rather to regulate the monthly cycle of hormone production necessary for her to become pregnant. Maturation of the follicle with its production of estrogen under the influence of FSH, the stimulation of LH release by this production of estrogen, the induction of ovulation by LH release, and the subsequent transformation of the follicle into a corpus luteum which produces progesterone, must occur in a precise and orderly fashion. The mere production of estrogen and progesterone, and the mere release of FSH and LH, are not sufficient. Fortunately, in most cases of "misfiring," the proper synchrony can be restored.

## Fertilization of the Egg in the Fallopian Tube

The goal toward which all of these processes lead is the fertilization of the egg by the sperm. This is a beautiful and moving event to observe under the microscope, and only recently have scientists come to understand fertilization well enough to duplicate it in a test tube and produce a normal baby.

Fertilization of the egg occurs in the widened region of the female's tube, called the ampulla. In most animals the egg will find sperm waiting when it arrives in the tube, because the period of sexual receptivity usually begins just before ovulation. Humans are the only animals in which there is no fixed relation between sexual intercourse and ovulation, and therefore our eggs may very well have to wait for the arrival of spermatozoa. The egg is capable of being fertilized only for a period of six to eight hours after ovulation. If it has to wait too long for sperm to arrive, all the effort that went into preparing the egg during the previous two weeks will have been in vain.

The number of sperm which actually reach the site of fertilization is terribly small when one considers the microscopic size of the sperm and the comparatively enormous volume of space within this region of the tube where the egg sits waiting. The actual contact of a sperm with the egg is governed mostly by chance.

For a sperm to enter and fertilize the egg, it must dig its way through several layers of protecting shields that surround it. All of these outside walls protecting the inner confines of the egg represent an impressive barrier to sperm penetration, and a sperm cannot break its way through these protective membranes without the aid of chemicals released from its warhead, the acrosome. The acrosome surrounds the front portion of the sperm, much like a battering ram. Chemicals released by the acrosome first dissolve the jellylike cumulus oophorus, enabling the sperm to pass through it and reach a tougher inner membrane, the zona pellucida. This very tough membrane represents perhaps the most formidable obstacle to sperm. To penetrate this barrier, the sperm cannot just haphazardly liberate chemicals, or the egg might be damaged. The attacking chemicals must remain closely bound to the surface of the sperm and cut an extraordinarily narrow slit in the membrane which allows only a single sperm to enter.

When this first sperm has successfully invaded the egg, a remarkable event takes place. The membrane which surrounds the egg fuses with the membrane of the sperm, and the sperm and the egg become one. The egg literally swallows the sperm as these two microscopic entities initiate the development of a new human being. At this moment the membranes surrounding the egg become transformed into a rigid barrier so impenetrable that other sperm, despite all the chemicals in their acrosomes, cannot possibly enter. Often many sperm can be seen attempting to enter the egg in competition with the one that made it first, but their efforts are totally in vain. Once the egg has been successfully penetrated by a single sperm, it shuts its walls so tightly that none of the followers can possibly get through.

Humans are relatively wasteful in their management of their sperm and eggs. If pregnancy does not occur in one month, it may occur in another. It's just that haphazard. However, in other animals the process is much more precise and careful. In the domestic hen, for example, spermatozoa are capable of living for four weeks in the female after deposit, and large numbers of eggs are fertilized as they pass through the hen during the next month. In bats, sexual intercourse takes place only in the autumn, and the animals then go to sleep for the winter. Three or four months later, when they wake up, the females finally ovulate, and the sperm which have been stored successfully during the entire winter are quite capable of fertilization despite their long period of waiting in the female. The honey bee is perhaps the most careful utilizer of sperm in the animal kingdom. After one nuptial flight with a male, the queen bee has a sufficient supply of spermatozoa to last for several years. She rations out one or two spermatozoa for each egg that is to be fertilized, and thus can produce millions of offspring over a period of years with the sperm received from one episode of intercourse. In certain spiders, the male deposits fewer than ten sperm in the female at the time of intercourse, but each of these carefully rationed sperm (think of the hundreds of millions of sperm deposited in the human female with each sexual act), each of these spider spermatozoa, is a jewel. The female may save them for up to a year to fertilize her eggs. The reproductive act seems to be efficient and precise in almost all members of the animal kingdom other than humans. The human reproductive mechanism is clearly developed in such a way that fertilization of the egg is not its only purpose.

EARLY DEVELOPMENT OF THE FERTILIZED EGG

Over the next three days the fertilized egg first divides into two cells, and then each of those cells divides to make four cells; finally each of those cells divides again to make eight cells. By the time this stage is reached, the embryo is ready to be passed from the tube into the womb, where it implants, and then goes on to develop over the next nine months into a baby. Once the pregnancy has been properly established in the womb, the embryo itself begins to make a hormone called chorionic gonadotropin, which stimulates the corpus luteum to keep making progesterone for the next three months.

The presence of chorionic gonadotropin signifies an established pregnancy, and is thus the basis for almost all of the routine pregnancy tests. When the doctor samples the patient's urine or blood and checks for pregnancy, he or she is really checking for the presence of chorionic gonadotropin. If it is present, then the patient is told that the pregnancy test is positive. Since previous methods of analyzing this hormone were not very sensitive, the diagnosis of pregnancy could not be made with certainty until about four weeks after the missed period. However, with sophisticated modern methods pregnancy can be diagnosed even before the woman realizes that she has missed her period.

ARE SPERM REALLY NECESSARY?

The egg may actually be activated into developing a new individual even though sperm did not penetrate it, and true fertilization hasn't taken place. This is popularly thought of as cloning, although the scientific word for it is parthenogenesis. For example, if one simply pricks a frog's egg with a needle, it will often undergo development just as though it had been fertilized by a sperm, and develop into a free-swimming, normal-appearing tadpole. These tadpoles have the genetic constitution of their mothers, but, unlike "clones," they are not identical twins to their mothers. Usually these tadpoles die and do not develop into mature frogs, but occasionally such "cloned" tadpoles do develop into mature and outwardly normal frogs. Thus in frogs the influence of the penetrating spermatozoa in activating division of the egg and the formation of a new individual may be purely mechanical.

Another example of this "cloning" in nature is the Amazon molly, a curious species of fish in which there are no males at all. The female fish mates with males of a different species and the spermatozoa cannot truly fertilize the egg but rather simply penetrate the egg and activate it. These activated eggs develop into completely normal female adult Amazon mollies. Since these fish did not result from normal fertilization, one would guess that they have half the proper number of genes and chromosomes. They do in fact have a normal number of genes, but both sets come from the mother. Although test-tube fertilization with sperm in humans is now a reality, there are no reliably documented cases of human parthenogenesis, or "clones."

Parthenogenesis is a common mode of reproduction in some insects, such as the honey bee. Drones are produced from the female's egg in the absence of any sperm. However, workers and queen bees are produced by proper fertilization with sperm. Experiments similar to pricking the frog egg with a needle have been attempted in mice and rabbits with development occasionally progressing as far as halfway through pregnancy. However, there are no successful reports of parthenogenesis resulting in a normal, live birth in any animals higher than the frog.

A form of parthenogenesis utilizing two eggs rather than one, and no sperm, has recently been developed. Studies indicate that sperm are not absolutely necessary for fertilization; it is simply more convenient to have them. In the laboratory, two eggs can be used to fertilize each other without the need for sperm. Such individuals would be completely normal genetically, and all would be females.

Reproductive biologists have suggested that there might be somewhere in human or mammalian populations an individual who developed spontaneously by parthenogenesis. Such an individual would of course be female, and would resemble her mother very closely, but there would be no other telltale features. We will discuss this subject in more detail in the chapter on test-tube babies and cloning. For the moment it is touched upon to show that as we come to understand the miracle of fertilization better, we may develop more futuristic methods of solving the problems of infertile couples.

# ·2·

# The Male's Role

## How the Testicles Work

### TEMPERATURE REGULATION

A normal male has two testicles, side by side. The testicles, or testes, are located in the scrotum, or scrotal sac. The scrotal sac consists of an outer layer of skin and several inner linings. The testicles are located in these exteriorized sacs because they do not function well inside the warm environment of the body. By residing outside of the body in a separate sac, the testes remain at a temperature about four degrees lower than the usual 98.6° F maintained in the rest of the body. The testicles are so sensitive to these four degrees of extra heat that if they were inside the body they would not be able to produce sperm.

The scrotum has a remarkably delicate temperature-regulating mechanism that keeps the temperature of the scrotal sac at 94° F at all times. Taking a cold shower causes the muscles of the scrotal sac to contract and pull the testes very close up against the body to conserve heat. On the other hand, when it is warm the scrotal muscles relax, and the testicles fall farther away from the body in order to cool off. This is an automatic reflex over which males have no control. In addition to this muscular thermal regulatory mechanism, there is a complicated network of arteries providing blood to the testes, and veins bringing blood away from the testes, which contract and dilate in accordance with external temperature so as to maintain just the right amount of blood flow to keep the testicles' temperature at 94° F. As we shall see later, alterations in this temperature-regulating mechanism are a common cause of male infertility.

### INTERNAL STRUCTURE OF THE TESTICLES

The testicle has two major functions. One is to make the male hormone, testosterone, which is responsible for the development of male sexual characteristics and male sexual behavior. The other is to produce spermatozoa, or sperm, capable of fertilizing the female's egg. The testicle consists of several hundred coiled microscopic tubules, called seminiferous tubules, in which the sperm are manufactured. These tubules converge and collect into a delta (like the mouth of a river) near the upper part of the testicle. This delta (called the rete testis) then empties through a series of five to seven very small ducts out of the testicle toward the vas deferens (Fig. 6). In between the microscopic seminiferous tubules which

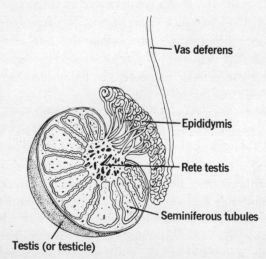

*Figure 6.* The Testicle.

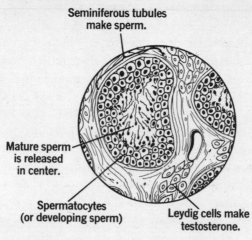

Seminiferous tubules
make sperm.

Mature sperm
is released
in center.

Spermatocytes
(or developing sperm)

Leydig cells make
testosterone.

*Figure* 7. Sperm and Hormone Production.

manufacture the sperm are clumps of cells (called Leydig cells) which make the male hormone, testosterone. These Leydig cells appear to be sprinkled like pepper throughout the substance of the testicle (Fig. 7).

Whereas sperm are carried out of the testicle into the vas deferens to be ejaculated at the time of orgasm, the male hormone manufactured by the Leydig cells is picked up by tiny veins coursing through the testicle. These tiny veins carry the male hormone into the circulation. It is because the male hormone drains into the circulation this way, rather than via the seminiferous tubules and vas deferens, that a man can undergo vasectomy (which means that his vas deferens is intentionally cut for sterilization) without altering his hormone production or sexual drive.

The Leydig cells, which produce the male hormone, are remarkably sturdy. It is very difficult for any sort of illness or disease to interfere with an adequate production of male hormone. However, the seminiferous tubules which manufacture sperm are extraordinarily delicate, and the slightest imperfection or generalized illness, such as a simple flu virus, can hurt sperm production. That is why so many men suffer from fertility problems, and yet have no lack of virility.

HORMONAL REGULATION OF SPERM PRODUCTION

Both the production of testosterone (which accounts for male sex drive, beard, pubic hair, and other sex characteristics) and the production of sperm are regulated by hormones produced by the pituitary gland, which sits just underneath the brain. These pituitary hormones are in turn regulated by "releasing factors" produced by the most primitive area of the brain, called the hypothalamus. This primitive region of the brain stimulates the pituitary gland to produce and release the two hormones FSH (follicle-stimulating hormone) and LH (luteinizing hormone). These names were given to the pituitary hormones on the basis of what they do in the female. However, they are exactly the same hormones which in the male stimulate the function of the testicles. Without the pituitary gland and without the primitive region of the brain, the testes in the male and the ovaries in the female would shrivel up and cease to function.

In the male FSH helps to stimulate and maintain proper sperm production. LH stimulates and maintains production of the male hormone, testosterone. When luteinizing hormone stimulates the testicles, the testosterone thus produced tells the brain that there is enough male hormone around, thus turning off the brain's production of the releasing hormone. As the production of this releasing hormone is turned off, the pituitary gland gets the message and in turn makes less LH. Consequently, less testosterone is produced by the testicles. On the other hand, when the testosterone level drops too low, this tells the primitive region of the brain that there is not enough hormone around and stimulates the brain to produce more releasing hormone, which in turn stimulates the pituitary to make more LH, so that the testicles then produce more testosterone. The brain thus helps to regulate the amount of testosterone produced by the testes, and, in ways that are less clearly understood, helps also to regulate the production of sperm.

Men who have severely damaged testicles (or who have no testicles at all) have extremely high circulating levels of releasing hormone from the primitive brain (and thus high levels of LH and FSH from the pituitary). These pituitary hormones are responding to a deficiency in testicular production of hormone by reaching high levels in an effort to whip whatever testicular tissue exists into functioning at the maximum possible capacity. Many men with severely damaged testicles still have normal male hormone levels (and normal sexual drive) only because their brain and pituitary are pouring out enormous quantities of releasing hormone to drive what little testicular tissue they have to maximum production.

The way in which the brain regulates production of sperm and hormones for the testicles is so important that we might dwell on an interesting example of a patient of mine who was born with *no testicles* at all, and who underwent a successful testicle transplant from his identical twin brother. This patient originally did not undergo puberty when he went through his teens. He remained a eunuch while all of his classmates underwent the usual growth spurt and sexual development that occurs at puberty. Because of the absence of the male hormone testosterone, he had no pubic hair, he had no sexual drive, he had no voice change, and he had no growth spurt. However, the levels of FSH and LH production from his pituitary and releasing hormone production from his brain were extraordinarily high. Since there was no testosterone being produced (by virtue of the fact that he had no testicles), the brain was constantly being given the message that there was an inadequate amount of male hormone. Since the brain had no way of knowing that there were no testicles in this patient, it responded in the normally programmed fashion by making excessive amounts of releasing hormone in an effort to drive the testicles into greater hormone and sperm production. When we successfully transplanted a testicle into him (using microsurgical techniques that will be explained in more detail in subsequent chapters), he began to produce testosterone almost immediately. At that point his blood FSH and LH levels finally came down to normal. After thirty years this patient's brain was finally being given the message that there was an adequate amount of testosterone in the circulation. On the other hand, were it not for the releasing hormone produced by the primitive area of the brain, and the FSH and LH hormones produced by the pituitary, the transplanted testicle could never function.

## SPERM PRODUCTION—THE ASSEMBLY LINE

The testicles normally produce sperm at a phenomenal rate, so that sperm are ejaculated in seemingly extravagant numbers. Think of the unbelievable sperm wastage that seems required for male fertility. Out of perhaps 200 million sperm inseminated with one act of intercourse, only four hundred ever reach the vicinity of the egg, and only a single sperm has even a 15 percent chance in any given month of fertilizing the egg. Because male fertility in many respects is a simple numbers game which any bookie would understand, we will describe the various steps in the production of a sperm, and what factors, if any, influence the quantity of sperm produced.

All of the cells that eventually develop into normal sperm are called germ cells. The germ cells within the seminiferous tubules of the testes are lined up in an orderly array with the most primitive early cells lying along the outer edge and the more developed sperm moving toward the center. All of these cells are held in place and nourished by a sort of formless or shapeless nurturing cell called the Sertoli cell. The germ cell, or developing sperm, sits with its head imbedded within the membrane of this Sertoli cell. In the final phase of sperm production the sperm develops an oval head and a tail necessary for locomotion. When the product is complete, the mature spermatozoon is released from the Sertoli cell into the tubule and swept along toward the efferent ducts to make its escape, along with millions of others, from the testicle.

As sperm go through their development process they are passed along toward the center of the tubule as though on an assembly line. In fact, the comparison of sperm production to an assembly line is quite accurate, since the sperm are passed along from one stage of production to another at an absolutely unalterable speed of sixteen days for each stage of production. The sperm go through four and a half such stages of production. Thus the total time it requires to produce every sperm is about seventy-two days. Neither sickness, testicular damage, nor hormonal manipulation can alter this inexorable rate at which the individual spermatozoa are produced. If one can imagine an automobile assembly line with a slow, steady, unstoppable movement from one stage of production to progressively more complex stages of production until the final car comes out for inspection, then one will have a pretty good understanding of how sperm are produced, and indeed how sloppy the results can often be. In fact, one might speculate that one reason for the extravagant number of sperm produced by the testicles is that only a small percentage will actually have all their nuts and bolts in the right place.

A deficiency in sperm production does not result from a slowing down of the speed at which the developing sperm proceed along the assembly line. Rather, a deficiency in sperm production results from an absent worker, or a missing part at any one of the stages along the way. Sometimes the problem may be simply an inadequate number of the earliest precursors of sperm. If there are a deficient number of these early precursors, then the total number of sperm produced will be inadequate. Also, a specific hormone or enzyme necessary for the passage of sperm from one stage of production to the next may be absent; this is called a spermatogenic arrest. There is no treatment that can possibly increase the speed of sperm production. The only hope for improving sperm production is either to replace a missing part, or enzyme, or to increase the number of early sperm precursors from which the spermatozoa are formed.

A simple understanding of this concept should make the reader depressingly aware of how difficult it is to improve sperm production in a man with a low sperm count. Many patients have been treated in a haphazard and unscientific manner to improve the sperm count, and the majority of these regimens are of unproven value. That is why treatment of the female to maximize her fertility potential must never be neglected, since it is often more likely to be effective than trying to increase sperm production.

## THE REASON WE NEED SO MANY SPERM

Why do we need to produce so many sperm? Why should such an enormous number of sperm be needed simply to fertilize one egg? How could nature be so wasteful and so stupid as to place a requirement upon us to overproduce vast numbers of these little creatures when only one is necessary to make a baby? Why should there be so many obstacles in the female genital tract which make it mandatory for a large number of sperm to be wasted just so that one will make it? Wouldn't it be easier if nature had provided us a simple little test tube in which one sperm could be mixed with one egg and a baby thus formed?

There are a number of reasons for this overproduction. First, the time during which an egg in the female can be fertilized after it is ovulated is brief, less than eight hours. Therefore, it must be fertilized promptly after its release from the ovary. This requires the continuous presence of a reasonable number of fresh sperm in the tube. It is therefore necessary for a much larger number of sperm to be available lower down in reservoir regions of the womb, to be continuously and slowly released upward. Another reason for the obstacles which the sperm must overcome is that intercourse is not a sterile process and the female genital tract must be protected against infection. The same immune and physical barriers which only allow a few lucky sperm to gain access to the egg also protect the female against invasion by bacteria. Finally it may be that sperm production is such a complicated biological process that there will be many defective products, again as on the automobile assembly line, and only the true "gems" are allowed access all the way to the egg.

### THE TESTICLES' PRODUCTION OF FEMALE HORMONE

Before we leave the testicles and explain the remarkable transport mechanism that allows these eager sperm to exit from the male's genitals and get their crack at the egg, we should emphasize that just as the female produces some male hormone (which is actually necessary for her sexual drive and hair growth), the male also makes some female hormone, estrogen. Remember that the stimulating hormones from the primitive region of the brain and the pituitary (FSH and LH) are the same in men and women. Furthermore, the male testicle and the female ovary each produce both male and female hormone. All that differs between men and women is that the testicle produces more male hormone, and the ovary produces more female hormone. When this delicate balance is ever so slightly upset, fertility may be compromised, without any other obvious effect.

## How Sperm Reach the Ejaculate

### LEAVING THE TESTICLES

After the completed spermatozoa are released into the seminiferous tubule, they flow along it toward the area called the rete testes, which is like a river delta near the upper edge of the testicle. Sperm are pushed along the seminiferous tubule toward this exit point by contractions of very delicate muscle fibers. The sperm do not move on their own. After they exit from the testicles, sperm are transferred into an amazing structure called the epididymis. The epididymis is a twenty-foot-long tube of microscopic size (one three-hundredth of an inch in diameter) which runs back and forth in loops like a strand of spaghetti, but which actually traverses a distance of only one and one-half inches. It transfers sperm from the testicle to the vas deferens, the male sperm duct. Imagine a twenty-foot-long spaghetti strand placed on a one-foot-long serving dish. At first such a plate would appear to be filled with many different strands of spaghetti. Similarly, with its multiple curves and convolutions the epididymis appears to be a large number of tubules, but it is actually just one very long tiny tubule.

It takes the sperm about twelve days to travel the entire twenty-foot journey through the winding length of the epididymis into the vas deferens. Sperm are propelled along this highly contorted microscropic tunnel by frequent contractions of its thin muscular wall. Most of the sperm are then stored at the end of the epididymis near where it joins the vas deferens. Here the sperm await their call to be rushed through the vas deferens and ejaculated at the time of orgasm.

## WHAT HAPPENS TO SPERM IN THE EPIDIDYMIS?

The epididymal tubule is not just a bridge between the testicle and the sperm duct. Sperm which leave the testicle are still not capable of fertilization. They must pass through the epididymis, the final tuning and inspection station of the assembly plant, before they obtain their ability to move in a straightforward direction with sufficient velocity to fertilize the female egg. If sperm were to be captured either from the testicle or from the beginning region of the epididymis, before the twenty-foot-long journey to the vas deferens, and used for artificial insemination of the wife, there would be no chance of pregnancy occurring. Only the sperm that reach the end of the epididymis, waiting to be released through the vas deferens upon orgasm, are maximally capable of fertilization. About half of the sperm located midway along the journey to the vas deferens are capable of fertilization. However, none of the sperm located in the earliest regions of the epididymis just after their exit from the testicle are capable of fertilization. During this seemingly endless journey through the winding turns of the epididymis, the sperm mature their structure and develop their incredible swimming ability.

Sperm motility is probably the most important determinant of the male's fertility. The sperm inside the testicle can only vibrate their tails weakly and barely wriggle around. Sperm from the beginning regions of the epididymis can swim, but only in circles. Unidirectional, straightforward swimming is only achieved by sperm that have traversed a good portion of the epididymis. In looking at the semen analysis of an infertile male, it is not only the percentage of sperm that are motile that counts, but also the quality of that motility. Sperm that swim in a curve are not capable of fertilization.

Sperm remain fresh and alive in the epididymis for a period of less than a month. Old age comes quickly to a little sperm, and if it has to sit around for a month in the epididymis waiting to be ejaculated, it will be of no use. This does not mean that the man who has intercourse only once a month need not fear an unwanted pregnancy. There are still fresh sperm arriving every day that upon ejaculation will be capable of fertilizing. However, a man who has an ejaculation only once a month will have a much higher percentage of dead, ineffectual sperm in his ejaculate, despite having a higher overall number of sperm stored up.

Although this would seem to be a rather short life span for the little creatures, it should be remembered that once they are deposited in a specimen jar, they are capable of living only for two to six hours. If they make it into the female genitals before that period has passed, they are capable of surviving for two to four days.

### THE FLUID THAT SQUIRTS THE SPERM OUT

Most of the fluid in the ejaculate does not come from the testicle, the epididymis, or the sperm duct. That is why vasectomy results in no change in the ejaculate aside from the absence of sperm. During sexual intercourse, the epididymis and vas deferens muscles contract powerfully and propel the sperm through the vas deferens along an eight-inch journey up and out of the scrotal sac into the abdomen and finally to the ejaculatory duct, which sits just in front of the bladder (Fig. 8). The ejaculatory duct empties into the urethra, the canal inside the penis that carries the ejaculate out of the body.

Most of the fluid comes from the seminal vesicles and the prostate gland. The seminal vesicles, located behind the bladder, expel their fluid very forcefully behind the sperm, pushing it into the urethra. The first portion of the ejaculate thus contains most of the sperm. The second portion is from the seminal vesicles, which contract violently and account for most of the ejaculatory fluid. At this time the internal sphincter of the bladder clamps down powerfully to prevent the semen from accidentally going backward into the bladder. At the same time it prevents urine from leaking forward out of the bladder. The external sphincter, which sits just in front of the ejaculatory duct, then opens up and allows the ejaculate to enter the holding area just near the base of the penis, the bulbous urethra. Finally the very powerful muscle bulbous urethra contract and squirt the ejaculate out of the penis with remarkable force. This highly coordinated symphony of complicated muscular contractions that propel the sperm from the epididymis all the way up through the abdomen and out the penis is what the male subjectively feels as orgasm.

Since the initial portion of the ejaculate contains the highest concentration of sperm, the patient who has been asked to collect semen for analysis will have an abnormally low reading if the first squirt is missed. The withdrawal method of contraception is relatively ineffective, for the same reason.

The volume of ejaculate is quite variable from person to person and from species to species. The human ejaculate is normally about one teaspoon, whereas the pig's ejaculate is close to a full pint. The amount of fluid needs to be sufficient to bathe the cervix

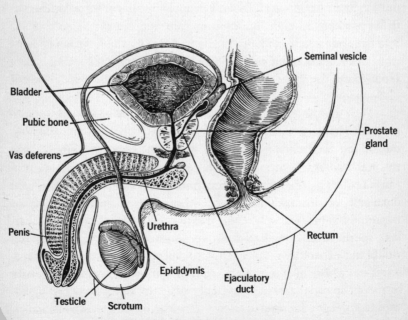

Figure 8. The Male Reproductive Organs (side view).

(the opening of the womb) with sperm so that they are not just left to die in the recesses of the vagina. Some otherwise fertile men may have a low ejaculate volume despite a normal sperm count. Their apparent infertility results from their sperm not really hitting the target, the woman's cervix.

It is clear that many of the complicated fluids secreted by the prostate gland, the urethral glands, and the seminal vesicles are not really necessary, except to provide a vehicle for sperm into the vagina. Though researchers have tried diligently to discover a role for the complex chemical constituents of this highly odoriferous fluid which carries the sperm into the vagina, they have not been terribly successful in their efforts. In fact, dilute solutions of salt water appear sometimes to be better for sperm than the semen in which they are naturally bathed at the time of ejaculation. The major function of the semen appears to be activation of the otherwise resting epididymal sperm at the time of ejaculation, and the provision of a suitable though very transient environment for them during the brief moment of transition from the man's vas deferens to the woman's vagina.

## How Many Sperm Do We Need?

Why does the male need so many millions of sperm when only one ever fertilizes the egg? We know that only four hundred sperm out of the 200 million normally ejaculated into the female ever reach the fallopian tube, and only forty ever get anywhere near the egg. The "test-tube" babies that have been made in England by mixing sperm from the husband with an egg taken from the wife require fewer than one million sperm. However, if only one million sperm were ejaculated into a normally fertile female, we would not expect a very great likelihood of pregnancy. There is a series of barriers in the female genitals that the spermatozoa must surmount in order to reach the egg. It is the difficulty of this passage to the egg that makes such a large army of sperm necessary. In a test tube these barriers don't exist, and indeed test-tube fertilization may be one solution on the horizon for men with very low sperm counts. But there are practical and less exotic solutions for the majority of couples in whom a low sperm count is discovered.

There are many unscientific pronouncements about how many sperm are needed for the man to be fertile. Every time one tries to define a lower limit of "normal" for sperm count, one always finds. some men who are demonstrably fertile, having impregnated their wives, but who have sperm counts which are lower than "normal." Twenty years ago, any man with a sperm count of less than sixty million sperm per cc was considered to be infertile. Such a figure would include over 40 percent of American men, when clearly not that many are infertile. Most doctors now recognize twenty million sperm per cc as the lower limit which divides fertile from infertile men. Yet despite these revised guidelines it is still very common to find pregnancies in couples where the man's sperm count is consistently less than twenty million sperm per cc.

In a recent exhaustive study by Professor Emil Steinberger of the University of Texas, two thousand fertile men requesting vasectomy underwent sperm counts prior to the vasectomy. Twenty-three percent of these fertile men had counts under twenty million sperm per cc and 11.7 percent had sperm counts under ten million sperm per cc. Only 43 percent of these men had sperm counts over sixty million sperm per cc. When more than 10 percent of a normal, fertile male population have exceedingly low sperm counts (less than ten million sperm per cc), it is very difficult to say what is normal and what is not. Yet surely common sense would suggest that men with such low sperm counts must have more difficulty impregnating their wives than men with higher sperm counts, and this is true: there is a significant decline in the likelihood of impregnation when the man's sperm count is below twenty million sperm per cc, and the greatest difficulty with impregnation occurs in partners where the man's sperm count is under ten million sperm per cc.

If the sperm count of the male is consistently below ten million sperm per cc, it is probably a major factor in the couple's infertility, but it does not rule out the reasonable possibility of pregnancy. In infertile couples where the husband's sperm count is five to ten million sperm per cc, 50 percent may achieve pregnancy despite long periods of prior infertility merely by full treatment of the wife. When the husband's sperm count is higher, the pregnancy rates with treatment of the wife increase to 80 percent. The treatment of the wife is more likely to be successful the higher the husband's sperm count.

Substantially encouraging pregnancy rates of 25 percent can be achieved in the worst possible group, where the husband's sperm count is below five million sperm per cc, merely by maximum treatment of the wife. Usually such a couple does not have such good fortune, because they are immediately referred to a urologist for treatment of the male's problem, and any further evaluation and treatment of the wife is deferred unless the husband's sperm count can be brought up to the more reasonable ranges of more than twenty million to more than sixty million sperm per cc. Since this achievement is very difficult in the male, very often these couples go without any treatment despite the fact that the most reliable way to treat a low sperm count in the majority of cases is to evaluate and treat the wife, who may have a contributory problem.

There is clearly no such thing as a "normal" sperm count, nor is there such a thing as an absolutely fertile or an absolutely infertile pattern of ovulation in the female. The fertility potential of both the husband and the wife are relative conditions, and in cases where the husband's low sperm count is untreatable, the greatest hope for success is in treating any subtle problems found in the wife. Nonetheless, if the husband's sperm count can be raised to higher levels, then the treatment of the wife is more likely to be successful. The treatment of only the husband or only the wife is a misconception that may result in no conception.

The problem of sometimes overemphasizing the detrimental effects of a low sperm count, to the neglect of the wife, is an interesting turnabout. Several decades ago the male's contribution to infertility was underplayed, and most infertility was improperly blamed completely on the female. During the last ten or fifteen years, appropriate attention has been called to the fact that the male's sperm count can be an important contributor to the problem of infertility. But in the process, the wife's role has become incorrectly undervalued.

A patient came into my office recently with a very worried look on his face. His wife had been seen by a gynecologist over the last year and a half because of their inability to achieve pregnancy, and the gynecologist, without even obtaining a sperm count from the husband, told the wife that the husband must be infertile, because he couldn't find any reason for the wife not to have gotten pregnant. This information resulted in tension between the two of them that reduced their frequency of intercourse from three times a week to once every two weeks, certainly not a help to their goal of getting pregnant. The problem created by the mismanagement of their infertility problems led to a crescendo of tension, with the husband begging for an early appointment to see what could be done about solving his problem. My secretary informed him that I would like to evaluate both the husband and the wife at the same time, and he explained to her, "No, no, you don't understand. She has already been evaluated and she is all right. It's me, it's my problem." My secretary finally convinced him that getting pregnant is the couple's problem, and we evaluated both partners.

After I did the husband's semen analysis and came into the room to greet them, he looked at me with extraordinary tension and asked, "Okay, what's the verdict?" His total sperm count was ninety-five million sperm per cc, certainly a very high sperm count. However, in questioning the wife we found that her periods had been regular until age sixteen, when they began to become very painful, and we also learned that she menstruated every nineteen to twenty days. She had slightly hairy arms, hair on her toes, and a few hairs on her breasts, all possible signs of an elevated testosterone level and poor ovulation. With a sperm count in the range of her husband's, I assumed that there would be an excellent chance of achieving pregnancy simply by treating the wife. Several months later, after treatment of the wife's poor ovulation, she became pregnant.

Overattention to the husband's low sperm count can frequently end in disaster. I treated a couple recently who were lucky, but whose story illustrates how the inability to get pregnant is usually due not just to the male or the female partner, but rather to a combination of problems in each of them. This couple had been married for three years, and although they used no birth control measures, the wife did not get pregnant. In 1974, she was evaluated at a major medical school. Her history revealed that she had had normal twenty-eight-day menstrual cycles of four to five days' duration until 1971, when they began to become irregular, lasting up to forty-five or fifty days. She was told that she was "probably" ovulating and fertile, but that her husband's sperm count (only one count was performed) was a low fourteen million sperm per cc. The gynecologist advised her that her husband was the problem. So her husband went to see a urologist.

Despite the fact that a man's sperm count can vary from one day to another and that no conclusion should be based upon a single sperm count, the urologist also swiftly informed this man that he was infertile (without repeating the sperm count). He was begun on a course of male hormone, methyl testosterone, for two and one-half months. This resulted in no pregnancy.

A year later, having moved to another state, the wife was seen by another gynecologist, and the husband by another urologist. The husband was then placed on a different hormone, which normally stimulates the testicles to produce the male hormone testosterone. His sperm count remained unchanged. The urologist reexamined the husband and decided that he probably had a small varicocele, a network of dilated varicose veins commonly found in the left testicle. Operating to tie off a varicocele often results in an improved sperm count. The urologist performed this surgery, but there was still no improvement in the husband's sperm count. He was then placed on another hormone-stimulating drug. Again no improvement in his sperm count, and no pregnancy.

After six years of neglecting the wife, a reevaluation of her ovulatory activity demonstrated that although she did ovulate, she ovulated late in the month, the quality of her eggs at the time of ovulation was not optimal, and the sperm had a difficult time penetrating her sticky cervical mucus. The cause of these problems was an elevated level of the male hormone, testosterone. She was given other hormones to suppress the overproduction of male hormone. A few months later her male hormone production was reduced to the normal female level, and she was ovulating at the right time with good eggs. In addition, there was improved penetration of her husband's sperm into her now more liquid cervical mucus. Four months after the beginning of her treatment, she conceived, and nine months later she delivered a normal baby.

The point of discussing this couple's six-year saga is to demonstrate that infertility is rarely absolute or limited to one partner, and that overattention to the man's low sperm count often causes neglect of an easily treated problem in the woman. There is usually a relative inadequacy in both the husband and the wife. Though this husband's sperm count was in a somewhat low range, it was not amenable to therapeutic improvement. Yet the wife's relatively low fertility was treatable. Had she not been carefully reevaluated and treated, they never would have had a child, and the blame would have always been placed on her husband's low sperm count.

Sometimes when the husband is informed that his sperm count is in a low range, or indeed that he is sterile, his reaction is one of complete disbelief, anger, and fear that his manhood is under attack. He should not take this negative attitude. The production of sperm is quite a separate matter from sexual ability. Just recently I saw an infertile couple, and I had the unfortunate duty of telling the husband that his sperm count was not optimal. The patient was six feet eight inches tall and weighed 280 pounds. He was an enormous hulk of a man with muscles everywhere. He and his wife had been trying for one and a half years to achieve pregnancy and he felt quite certain that he was not at fault. He was a bit hostile and reluctant about coming into the office to take part in their evaluation. I trembled as he suddenly sat up in his chair (which was sinking somewhat under his weight) and said with about the meanest look I have ever seen, "What do you mean, my sperm ain't normal?"

I explained to him the physiology of the testes, and that his sperm count could relate partially to their failure to have a baby. I emphasized that this was a problem with both partners, rather than any one individual. He was really quite furious to hear all of this and insisted that it could only be his wife's fault. He explained to me that he ate a lot of meat and pork chops and was sure that he should therefore have a good sperm count. He elaborated that he had eaten fish a few nights before, and that perhaps this was the reason his sperm count was low, since he knew that fish was not as good for him as pork chops. I tried to explain to him that none of these factors was really relevant but agreed that several more sperm counts would be necessary to assess his true fertility potential since sperm counts can vary so much from one examination to the next. It was very difficult to communicate sensibly with this man, as his pride was terribly wounded by his incorrect association of sperm count with virility.

A final note of caution for the male who is worried about whether the barrenness of the marriage is the result of his low sperm count: sperm counts have an enormous intrinsic variability from month to month and through the years. You should beware of a urologist who is ready to try you on one form of medication or another (or surgery) without first obtaining an adequate number of semen analyses and working out an average sperm count so as to evaluate correctly the need for such therapy. In many cases where the sperm count is relatively low, the therapy available for attempting to raise it is somewhat speculative. This does not mean that efforts to raise the sperm count are not worthwhile. They are. However, they must not be undertaken until an adequate number of semen analyses have been performed to judge whether you really have a problem.

As a perfect example of the confusion and mental anguish often created by this normal variability in sperm count, I recently received a letter from a patient's wife, who appeared to be on the brink of despair. We had performed a successful vasectomy reversal on her husband. He had a normal sperm count of sixty million sperm per cc, but she had failed to obtain a detailed gynecological evaluation because her doctor told her she was "normal." When she failed to conceive, her husband obtained another sperm count which this time was much lower, twenty million sperm per cc. Her gynecologist again neglected to perform a careful evaluation of her fertility status but sent her husband to a local urologist who knew nothing about infertility. The urologist placed the husband on Cytomel, a thyroid preparation which twenty years ago was thought to stimulate sperm production but which has subsequently been discredited as a form of therapy for infertility. Shortly after this, the wife wrote me a frantic letter asking what to do.

I suggested that he stop taking the Cytomel before he developed thyroid complications, and that he get a series of three more sperm counts performed at different laboratories and at different times over the next several months. Without any treatment whatsoever, these subsequent sperm counts were all very high, over 100 million sperm per cc. The variability of sperm counts can be confusing and unsettling. She eventually became pregnant.

Most infertile couples represent a combination of problems in the wife and the husband, so the answer to the question of how many sperm are needed is not an absolute one. It appears that one of the major reasons for the extravagant numbers of sperm necessary to produce a single conception is the significant number of hurdles facing these sperm as they enter the female genitals on their way to the egg. Therefore it should not be surprising that one of the best ways of treating infertility related to low sperm counts is to lower those hurdles in the female and not neglect the opportunity to maximize the wife's fertility potential despite the fact that the husband may have what is considered to be a low sperm count.

# ·3·

# Figuring Out What's Wrong

## How Long Does It Take to Get Pregnant, or When Should We Begin to Worry?

Even for couples who have no infertility problems, pregnancy does not usually occur in the first or even the second month. When my wife and I decided to start our family, it took a full six months before she finally conceived. After each month passed with no pregnancy, we agonized, "What if we cannot have children?" On the other hand, we have friends with children who were not able to achieve pregnancy for many years and never even bothered to consult a doctor. So when should you begin to worry that you might not be able to have children? Is there a particular time beyond which you should fear that you may be infertile, and seek medical attention? All potential parents-to-be will need a little lesson in statistics from this section to understand the similarity between becoming pregnant and rolling dice. That's the only way you will know when to start worrying.

Getting pregnant is basically a game of odds. Some couples are simply likely to get pregnant sooner then others. If infertile couples had three hundred years in which to breed, it seems almost certain that eventually without any treatment most wives would become pregnant. But the usual breeding period for families is no more than fifteen years, so the odds need to be considerably improved. When a couple has waited as long as one or two years without achieving pregnancy they might seem infertile, and by the end of that time they would almost certainly be frantic. Yet many of these couples may not be infertile at all, but merely victims of statistical chance, having no less likelihood of pregnancy occurring with each given month than the couple that was fortunate enough to get pregnant at their first attempt.

What is the probability in any given month of a normal, fertile couple's achieving a pregnancy? I recently posed this question to several authorities on population. I was surprised to find that most of them considered it a very difficult question to answer with accuracy. Yet it is critically important to understand the natural incidence of pregnancy month by month in a fertile population, so that the couple having difficulty with conception can understand whether or not they really have a problem.

Studies in England as far back as the 1850s demonstrated that young women get pregnant sooner and more easily than older women. The incidence of infertility in women twenty-five years of age was 7 percent and the incidence of infertility in women thirty years of age was approximately 13 percent. At thirty-five years of age 20 percent of women were unable to have children. By age forty, 32 percent of women were unable to get pregnant.

Modern population studies show that about 40 percent to 50 percent of women achieve pregnancy within the first four months of trying. After two years about 9 percent of women still have not yet conceived. Are the 50 percent to 60 percent of women who are not yet pregnant after four months of trying any less fertile, or any less likely to achieve pregnancy in subsequent months, than those who have already been lucky enough to conceive? Are the 9 percent of women who have not conceived after two years a hard-core group with severe infertility problems, or do they just represent a statistical inevitability which may be erased with the next monthly cycle?

Think of fertility in these terms: if one were to flip a coin three times in a row, and land tails each time, he might think that on the next flip he would be more likely to land heads than tails. Of course this is not true. Each time the coin is flipped there is a fifty-fifty chance of its landing either heads or tails, regardless of the past history. To really understand the likelihood of conception with each passing month (and when a couple perhaps should start worrying), we must not be concerned too early by unsuccessful flips.

Modern studies have shown that with the most fertile population of patients (those who eventually went on to raise large families) there was only a 20 percent chance in any given month of the wife's becoming pregnant. If she was not pregnant after six months, the chance that she would become pregnant in the seventh month was still only 20 percent. This study also showed that for a fertile couple trying to achieve pregnancy, the more sex the better. The concept of abstaining for several days to make the sperm count higher may sometimes benefit men with very low sperm counts, but such an approach does not increase the fertility of a normally fertile couple. Studies of artificial insemination from Belgium have also shown that with each succeeding month the chance for pregnancy is no less in normal women who have not yet conceived than in those who were lucky enough to become pregnant in the very first month. This should be of some comfort to those couples whose fertility tests have been normal, but who simply have not yet achieved pregnancy.

The studies in Belgium began with 632 normally fertile women whose husbands had complete absence of sperm in their ejaculate. Very fertile donor sperm was used to inseminate each female just prior to ovulation each month until she became pregnant. In the first month 130 of the 632 women became pregnant (20.57 percent). In the second cycle 103 more women became pregnant (16.29 percent). In the third monthly cycle 81 more women became pregnant (12.81 percent). Thus a total of 49.67 percent of the 632 women starting in this series achieved pregnancy within the first three months. In the fourth month 54 more women became pregnant (8.54 percent). In the fifth month 40 women became pregnant (6.32 percent). By six months a total of

73 percent of the patients had become pregnant. It is at this point that the other 27 percent of the women might have been tempted to give up.

However, if we figure the percentage of pregnancies for each month only among the women who were trying to conceive that month, there is a strikingly constant probability (20 percent) of pregnancy each month. Of the 632 patients undergoing insemination in the first month, 130 became pregnant, 20.56 percent of those inseminated. Of the 502 remaining women inseminated in the second month, 103 became pregnant, or 20.47 percent. This left 399 women who underwent insemination in the third month. Eighty-one of them became pregnant—20.3 percent. However, this represented only 12.8 percent of the original 632 women. In the tenth month only 3 percent of the total women starting this program became pregnant, but the pregnancy rate among the women who were actually inseminated was still 20.21 percent. By that time there were only 94 women out of the original 632 who had not yet achieved pregnancy, yet in that month 19 women, or 20.21 percent, conceived. In the eighteenth month after the beginning of this study, 5 women (less than 1 percent of those originally entering the study) became pregnant. However, by that time only 23 women were remaining who had not yet achieved pregnancy, and the 5 who became pregnant that month represented 21.75 percent of those remaining.

Thus it would appear that even though the majority of fertile women become pregnant within the first six months of trying, and only a tiny minority require as long as eighteen months or two years to become pregnant, nonetheless we can see that with each succeeding month, each woman still has a 20 percent chance of becoming pregnant.

In these tests several patients did not achieve pregnancy until three years after beginning the program, but when these women came back to have their second child, many became pregnant within just a few months. In addition some women who had achieved pregnancy very early with their first child required a much longer time to become pregnant with the second child, despite no obvious change in their fertility. If the conception rate in any large group of women trying to achieve pregnancy in a given month is 20 percent, it is a mathematical certainty that a small number of them will not obtain their goal until several years have passed.

It all comes back to the simple example of flipping coins. The chances of landing heads on any given flip is of course 50 percent. That means that if one hundred players were to line up with their coins and flip them, only fifty would turn up heads the first go-around. That would leave fifty players left to flip coins again. Only twenty-five of the fifty would turn up heads the second time. That would mean that twenty-five players are left who had flipped their coins twice in a row and lost both times, even though they had a 50 percent chance with each flip of getting heads. If these twenty-five remaining players now all flip their coins again, only twelve of them are going to land heads on the third try. Only six of the remaining twelve who had consistently failed to flip heads on three tries would turn up heads finally on the fourth try. The remaining six might erroneously conclude that there is something wrong with their coin, even though it was mathematically inevitable that after four rounds six players would never have flipped heads. The biggest mistake these remaining six players could make would be to give up, thinking that the coins they are flipping are incapable of turning up heads.

Dr. Charles Westoff of Princeton University, using a similar mathematical approach, has worked out the probability of conception with each month for "fertile" couples of various ages (see Table 1). Once you figure out the monthly probability of conception, it is easy to compute the chances of a fertile couple's achieving pregnancy within six months, one year, or two years. For young women in their early twenties, the monthly probability of conception is generally between 20 percent and 25 percent. By four months about 50 percent of women in this age group will have achieved pregnancy (assuming a 20 percent chance with each month); about 94 percent will be pregnant within the first year. For women in their late twenties and early thirties, however, the probability of conception is somewhat lower, in the range of 10 percent to 15 percent each month. In such a group only about 70 percent to 85 percent will achieve pregnancy within the first year. However, those who have not become pregnant within the first year will still have the same 10 percent to 15 percent chance of becoming pregnant in each succeeding month. They should not give up simply because they did not become pregnant in the first year.

**Table 1. Likelihood of Pregnancy in
Fertile Women—How Long Should It Take?**

| AGE | PROBABILITY OF CONCEPTION PER MONTH | AVERAGE TIME TO CONCEPTION (MONTHS) | PROBABILITY OF CONCEPTION WITHIN A YEAR |
|---|---|---|---|
| Late 30s | 8.3% | 12 | 65% |
| Early 30s | 10% | 10 | 72% |
| Late 20s | 15% | 6.7 | 86% |
| | 20% | 5 | 93% |
| Early 20s | 25% | 4 | 97% |

For women in their early twenties—and presumed to be highly fertile—the monthly probability of conception is thought to be between 20 percent and 25 percent, in the absence of contraception.

For somewhat less fertile women, in their late twenties and early thirties, the monthly probability of conception is lower: between 10 percent and 15 percent. Around 72 percent to 86 percent conceive within a year.

This discussion of pregnancy rates in "normal" fertile women demonstrates that fertility is not an absolute, easily definable quality. Even in a group of women with uniformly normal fertility, many will have a long wait before they achieve their pregnancy. It is a simple mathematical inevitability.

So we come back to the old question "When should the couple begin to worry and when should they seek medical attention?" If we had three hundred years in which to breed, the majority of infertile couples would eventually have children without treatment. It is difficult to know whether a particular couple's conception probability per month is 20 percent, 15 percent, 10 percent, or 1 percent. The mere fact that a year has gone by without pregnancy does not necessarily signify that they have a problem. Seeing a doctor too soon can sometimes hinder rather than help.

I recently saw a couple who were on the verge of divorce because of an artificial schedule (that their doctor had suggested) of withholding intercourse until ovulation. They had been trying unsuccessfully for eight months to achieve pregnancy. Their doctor, who was a little bit out of date, insisted that they avoid all intercourse for the first two weeks of the monthly cycle, take basal body temperatures, and then methodically have intercourse exactly on the day that the woman's temperature went up. This advice not only created terrible tension in their sex life, but also succeeded in reducing their chances for pregnancy because once the temperature goes up (and ovulation has occurred), the chances of impregnation are considerably less than when intercourse is allowed prior to the temperature's going up. Thus without realizing it, rather then maximizing their chances for pregnancy, they were practicing a form of rhythm birth control. When I saw this couple four months later, my advice was to disregard all medical advice for the next six months, and just have a good sex life. She became pregnant after three months.

There is one ironic statistic to end this section which has to be a bit sobering to any fertility specialist. In a large population of fertile couples of all ages, about 60 percent will have achieved pregnancy by six months and 80 percent by twelve months. Only 90 percent of such fertile couples will have achieved pregnancy by one and a half years. This means that in the six-month period following the first year of no pregnancy, only 10 percent more women will conceive. But remember that this group represents a full 50 percent of the 20 percent of couples who did not achieve pregnancy in the first year. Thus half of those who had not achieved pregnancy by one year will have succeeded by a year and a half, *without any medical intervention whatsoever.* The physician who does nothing more than evaluate such couples and pat them on the head will achieve a 50 percent pregnancy rate in the next six months. Thus one cannot assume that the length of time a couple has been trying to have children specifically indicates their degree of fertility or infertility.

After guiding many couples through these agonizing months of waiting, this is my advice as to when to seek help: When the couple becomes so anxious and so worried that their happiness is at stake (which could occur after six months, or after one year) they should each have a full evaluation by a competent authority in the field of fertility. They should recognize, however, that if their evaluations by a competent physician are perfectly normal, their problem may simply be a mathematical one requiring nothing more than optimism and patience.

## Tests on the Male

### WHAT IS A SPERM COUNT?

One of the most important initial tests for evaluating a couple's infertility is the husband's sperm count. This is the single best method of determining to what degree the male partner is contributing to the couple's barrenness. No other test for evaluating the couple's infertility is quite so simple and important. Yet there are frequent errors in its performance, and a misinterpretation of the sperm count can have tragic consequences. For these reasons I shall explain in full detail the process of obtaining and interpreting the sperm count.

*What Are Sperm?* You should realize that what is commonly thought of as sperm is actually semen. Semen is the fluid ejaculated at the time of orgasm, and it may or may not contain sperm. It is impossible to tell by its appearance whether the semen contains sperm. For example, after a vasectomy a patient has perfectly normal ejaculation and notices no reduction in his semen. Yet, looking under the microscope, he will no longer see any sperm in his ejaculate.

Sperm (or spermatozoa) are microscopic creatures which look like tadpoles swimming about at a frantic pace back and forth in the semen. The thought of all these little animals scurrying about inside could give you the willies. Each sperm consists of a head which contains all of the genetic material of the father-to-be, and a tail which lashes back and forth at an incredible speed to propel the sperm along (Fig. 9). In the ejaculate of a fertile man there are millions of these sperm, and they usually move at a very rapid speed.

Upon first observation of sperm under the microscope, you can't help but be awestruck by the massive numbers, and by the rapid, gyrating pace of their movement. Perhaps more subtle and more important than the apparent frenzy of microscopic activity is

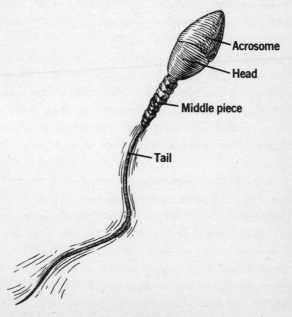

*Figure* 9. Sperm.

the purposefulness of the movements. Despite the fact that they are all moving in different directions (and so their motion appears to be haphazard and random), each one moves in a straight line with the accuracy of a guided missile. In a normal specimen each sperm that one fixes on goes straight across the field of the microscope without stopping, without turning around, without going in a pointless circle, and with no deviation from what appears to be a straight line. It is only the massive number of these sperm all mixed together and each going in different straight lines that superficially makes the motion appear random and haphazard.

*Obtaining a Proper Specimen.* The specimen must be collected properly, and brought into the laboratory for analysis within one to two hours. The laboratory must do an accurate numerical count as well as carefully observe the quality of the sperm. No matter how accurately the laboratory does the count and no matter how carefully and consistently the specimen is collected by the patient, there will be frequent variations in the total. For the patient to get any value out of the sperm count, it must be repeated at least three times over the course of several months.

Since intercourse will deplete the male temporarily of some sperm, it is important to abstain from intercourse for a few days prior to collecting the specimen. Otherwise a low value will be reported by the laboratory, and the husband may mistakenly conclude that he is sterile, even though his ejaculation just prior to obtaining the collection may have had a very large number of sperm.

On numerous occasions we have received frantic phone calls from wives worrying because their husband's sperm counts were reported as sterile by the laboratory. Frequently when the count is low we find that the couple had intercourse the night before. This can result in a reduction of the sperm count to one-third or less its normal level. Since the average American couple has intercourse two to three times a week, it has arbitrarily been felt that two to three days of abstinence prior to the performance of the sperm count will allow the count to reflect accurately how much sperm is delivered to the wife at the time of intercourse. If the couple has an unusually active sex life, then some sperm counts should be obtained without any period of abstinence. Then further sperm counts done after two to three days of abstinence will show whether any improvement can be derived from "saving it up."

If abstaining for two or three days prior to collection of the specimen results in a higher sperm count, it seems that abstaining for two weeks should bring the count up even more, and that abstinence should be a way of improving the husband's fertility. Unfortunately, abstaining for more than four or five days rarely results in any significant increase in the sperm count. If anything, those unused sperm that have been allowed to sit in the man's genitals for so long often have decreased potential for fertilization. The degree to which frequency of intercourse affects sperm production, sperm count, and fertility will be discussed in greater detail in another section on the timing of intercourse.

The semen specimen should be produced by masturbation, collecting the entire ejaculate in a wide-mouthed, clean collection jar that can be obtained from the laboratory. If the collection jar is not wide-mouthed, or if the specimen is obtained by coitus interruptus ("pulling out early"), it is easy to lose a small portion of the ejaculate. Notwithstanding the mess, this would result in great errors in the sperm count, since different portions of the ejaculate harbor different concentrations of sperm. In most men, the majority of sperm come out in the early portion of the ejaculate. Subsequent squirts after the first portion of the specimen usually contain very few sperm. Thus, if one were having a difficult time getting the bottle into the proper position and spilled an early portion of the ejaculate, the sperm count might turn out to be falsely low. Therefore, to obtain an accurate count, all of the ejaculation must be collected in one specimen container. Collection in a condom during intercourse is also not acceptable because most condoms have agents that kill sperm.

Having properly collected the semen specimen for analysis, the patient must bring it into the laboratory and have it examined within two hours. Though the sperm may live for up to a month within the male's reproductive system, and may live for two to four days in the female's system, they can live in the specimen collection jar for only two to five hours. If the analysis of the specimen is delayed more than two hours by late delivery to the laboratory or by inattention once the specimen reaches the laboratory, a large proportion of sperm may have died off or lost a good deal of their motility.

*How Many Sperm?* The two most important aspects of the sperm count are the actual numerical concentration of sperm per cubic centimeter and the motility of the sperm, that is, the speed and the quality of the movement. The number of sperm in the ejaculate is determined by looking at a tiny but measured portion of it in a counting chamber under a microscope. The laboratory technician will actually count each sperm in a given number of boxes that represent a specific volume of fluid. He or she can then calculate the total number of sperm in the ejaculate. If the count is thirteen million sperm per cc, a relatively low count, the technician will have counted only thirteen sperm within five boxes. If the count is 100 million sperm per cc, a very high count, the technician will have counted one hundred sperm in those five boxes.

*Motility of the Sperm.* More important than the quantity of sperm is the quality and activity of those sperm. After the specimen has been counted, the technician will observe the sperm under the microscope to determine what percentage of all the sperm seen in any microscopic field are actually moving and what percentage are not moving. There will always be a certain number of dead, nonmotile (nonmoving) sperm in the ejaculate. These nonmotile sperm are incapable of fertilization. Only the moving sperm are capable of entering the cervical mucus of the wife and ultimately reaching and penetrating the egg. After the percent motility is determined (that is, the percentage of moving sperm), the technician will observe and record the quality of that motion.

There are four types of sperm movement. *Grade I* motility means that the sperm are only wiggling sluggishly in place and making very little, if any, forward progression. These are pathetic vibratory-type motions that get the sperm nowhere. Such sperm are incapable of fertilizing the egg. *Grade II* motility means that the sperm are moving forward, but either the speed is very slow or they do not move in a straight line, instead veering off in a curve. Normally sperm have a remarkable propensity for maintaining straightforward motion. Sperm that cannot hold their course are incapable of fertilization. Some sperm go forward a little and then, instead of continuing undaunted, stop and reverse themselves. Such sperm will simply never make it in the ferocious arena of the female genital tract. *Grade III* sperm are able to move at a reasonable speed with straightforward progress and accurate homing. *Grade IV* sperm advance straight ahead also, but at an extraordinarily rapid speed. Grade III and Grade IV sperm are usually capable of fertilization. Grades I and II sperm generally are not.

*The Amount of Semen.* Most men ejaculate one-half teaspoon to one full teaspoon of semen (2.5 cc to 5 cc). There are a few men who have very low ejaculate volumes of less than a fifth of a teaspoon, and who may mistakenly think they have a very low amount of sperm. However, such men often have a very high concentration of sperm in that low volume. On the other hand, some patients may have a very high volume of ejaculate, well over a teaspoon. Such patients may have an adequate amount of sperm production but a low sperm concentration because the sperm are all diluted in such a relatively large amount of fluid; they may think that they are making a lot of sperm because of their high ejaculate volume when in fact they have a relatively low concentration. The total number of sperm ejaculated into the vagina is probably not as important as the concentration of sperm. Very large ejaculate volumes can be detrimental because a smaller concentration of sperm gets in contact with the wife's cervix and therefore a smaller number of sperm are able to attempt the arduous journey upward toward the egg.

In certain cases there may be no ejaculate whatsoever because all of the patient's sperm and seminal fluid are being ejaculated backward into the bladder rather than forward out of the penis.

This is a condition caused frequently by diabetes or by past surgery. In addition, certain patients on medication to control high blood pressure may have backward ejaculation of sperm into the bladder as a side effect of the medication. Such a patient may mistakenly believe that he is making no sperm at all whereas in truth he may be making large amounts of sperm. They are simply not getting out.

*The Appearance of the Semen—Liquid or Jelly?* Within a minute of ejaculation, the semen should normally coagulate into a tapiocalike gel. This change is referred to as clumping. The sperm cannot be adequately counted or examined while the semen is in this coagulated blob. The main function of clumping is probably to prevent early leakage of sperm out of the vagina. Within ten to thirty minutes after ejaculation, the blob should again liquefy.

Failure of sperm to reliquefy could indicate subtle infections of the prostate and seminal vesicles, but sometimes it is simply a normal variant, and subsequent semen collections on different days might present no problem. Failure of the semen to liquefy often leads to all sorts of false notions of infertility. Sometimes the patient is told that it means that the husband is allergic to himself and that his sperm are being attacked by his own antibodies.

An example of the foolishness of worrying about persistent coagulation (or nonliquefaction) of the semen is a patient who was recently referred to me with long-term infertility blamed on the persistent clumping of his semen (supposedly caused by an immune reaction). He and his wife had been trying to get pregnant for the last ten years. By the time that their appointment with me was made, the wife had finally been seen by a superb gynecologist, who found that she not only did not ovulate every month, but that she ovulated late and that her cervical mucus was too thick. The failure of her husband's sperm to penetrate her cervical mucus thus had been blamed incorrectly on his clumping problem. The gynecologist placed the wife on proper treatment. Just before the couple's appointment to see me, I received a telephone call from the wife saying that after ten years she had finally become pregnant without even entering my office. Clearly the failure of her husband's sperm to penetrate her cervix and enter her womb was due to a disturbance in her mucus, and a problem with ovulation, rather than to his clumpy semen.

*Sugar and Chemicals in the Semen.* There are a few tests performed on the semen itself, for sugar content, alkalinity, volume, and ability to coagulate and reliquefy. It appears that the only function of the complex, smelly chemistry of the semen is to deliver the sperm directly to the female cervix, and the function of this transporting fluid is indeed brief. Once secure within the cervical mucus, the sperm are safe. However, the sperm that don't make it into the cervical mucus will find that the fluid of the ejaculate is actually a hostile environment after several hours. The sperm appear to be relatively safe in the vas deferens and epididymis prior to ejaculation, and thereafter have a decent prospect for survival only after they penetrate the cervical mucus of the wife. It is in the precarious moment when the sperm are ejaculated into the vagina that time is of the essence. The semen's alkalinity protects against the acid in the vagina. The gelatinlike blob prevents early leakage out of the vagina, and the sugar provides instant energy for locomotion. The fluid of the ejaculate is not really designed to keep the sperm alive for very long, but only to get them on their way as quickly as possible into the cervical mucus.

*The Shape of the Sperm.* The final portion of the semen analysis is the microscopic examination for morphology, or structure, of the sperm. In a normal specimen as many as 30 percent of the spermatozoa may have abnormal structure (Fig. 10). There is no relationship between abnormal sperm and abnormal pregnancy. Abnormally shaped sperm cannot fertilize the egg. The normal sperm has an oval head with a long tail. Abnormally shaped sperm may have either a very large round head, or an extremely small, pinpoint head. They may have a thin, tapering appearance as compared with the thicker, oval appearance of a normal sperm head. They may even have two heads and look like Siamese monsters.

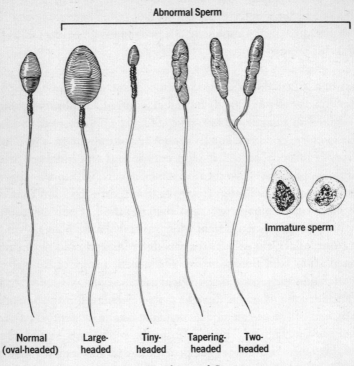

*Figure 10.* Abnormal Sperm.

The sperm may be bent at the neck and misshapen, and the tails may have kinks and curls in them. None of these horrifying-looking sperm (which are present in large numbers even in a normal ejaculate) is indicative of any genetic problem. However, such abnormally shaped sperm are not capable of fertilization.

There is a strong relationship between structure of the sperm and their motility. In general, abnormally shaped spermatozoa exhibit poor motility and normally shaped spermatozoa exhibit good motility. One advantage of checking the structure is that if the specimen is more than two hours old and its motility is therefore difficult to interpret, the structure is another measurement which may help to determine what percentage of the sperm are actually capable of fertilization. Sometimes immature sperm that do not even have tails can be seen in the ejaculate, representing an inadequacy in sperm production at the final stages of the assembly line. On the other hand, sometimes very vigorously moving tails that appear to exhibit good forward progression can be seen without any head on them at all. Again, such sperm, or half-sperm, are incapable of fertilization. The normal sperm has a head with an oval shape, no crooked bend at the neck, and a straight, long, tapering tail. If one looks at the sperm found in the wife's cervical mucus shortly after intercourse, it is rare to find abnormally shaped sperm, even though the husband's semen analyses may have demonstrated a large number of such abnormal sperm. The female cervical mucus tends to filter out the sperm that are misshapen and that have poor motility.

*The Postcoital Test—Sperm Invasion.* Although the sperm count is the single most accurate method of determining the male's fertility potential in the marriage, the ultimate benefit of a normal sperm count is to have a rapid and massive penetration of the wife's cervical mucus by the freshly ejaculated sperm. One way of checking this is to do a postcoital test on the wife, which is a sort of sperm count performed on the wife's cervical mucus after intercourse. If a large number of healthy, motile sperm are seen in the wife's cervical mucus after intercourse, it is a very good sign. Within two to five minutes of ejaculation, large numbers of sperm should have already entered the cervical mucus. Since the ejaculate has not even liquefied from its initial coagulation yet, this would indicate that sperm are able to gain quick access to the cervix and do not need to wait for liquefaction.

The difficulty with the postcoital test, despite its obvious functional importance, is that there is only a very short, precise interval during every month when a woman's cervical mucus is of the proper physical texture to permit sperm invasion. During the entire rest of the month, her cervical mucus represents a solid barrier to sperm penetration. Thus, if the postcoital test is not done at exactly the right time of the month, it may give a false impression that the husband's sperm is inadequate. Indeed, the usual cause for a poor postcoital test is improper timing of the test on the wrong day of the month, rather than any problem with the husband's sperm. Furthermore, in some women even this short interval during which the cervical mucus is sufficiently fluid to allow sperm penetration may not occur, and that may indeed be their fertility problem. Thus a sperm count must be performed on the husband on at least three occasions, and complemented by a microscopic analysis of the wife's cervical mucus after intercourse (only at the right interval during the month), in order to determine accurately the relative fertility of the male partner.

MEDICAL HISTORY

*Mumps in the Testicles.* After the sperm count, the most important test on the infertile man is the simplest and least expensive: the history and physical examination. There are no remarkable clues in the medical histories of most infertile men, but occasionally there is something. Mumps is a good example. In childhood, mumps does no harm to the testicles. But in adulthood, it is a vicious disease which causes swelling and pain in one or both testicles. In patients who recover fertility after adult mumps, progress is very slow.

I saw a man recently who had had a severe case of mumps involving the testicles when he was eighteen years of age. He was in the army at the time and his semen analysis performed shortly after recovery from the mumps demonstrated no sperm at all. He was told at the time that he would be permanently sterile. Three years later he got married and informed his wife that unfortunately they would not be able to have children. She accepted this with resignation but three months later turned up pregnant. The patient was furious, but his wife insisted that she had been loyal to him, so he decided to get another sperm count. This time his sperm was completely normal, in the range of forty million to sixty million sperm per cc with 80 percent motility. When people recover from mumps of the testicles, it generally takes more than a year, and sometimes as long as three to four years. So hope should not be given up too early, as it may take the testicles an extraordinarily long time to recover from such infections. Nothing medical science could offer would have been of any use to this patient, but luck and time were on his side.

*Scrotal Swelling.* A boy anywhere from several years of age up until the late teens or early twenties may have a sudden swelling of the testicle on one side which is terribly painful and which is not associated with the mumps. This can be caused by epididymitis, an infection of the epididymis best treated with antibiotics, or it can be caused by torsion, whereby the testicle twists on its own cord that attaches it to the body. This twisting causes a sudden interruption of blood flowing to the testicle and blood returning back from the testicle. The testicle swells up dramatically and becomes intensely painful. Most but not all cases of sudden acute testicular swelling in males under the age of twenty are caused by torsion. Most cases over the age of thirty-five are caused by epididymitis.

If antibiotics are not given promptly to a man who develops sudden epididymitis, he is likely to develop obstruction in the epididymis as it heals, and his sperm will be unable to get out. On the other hand, if a child with torsion does not undergo an immediate operation to untwist his testicle, over the next three months the swollen, painful testicle will shrink into a little pea-sized lump. The testicle will have died and withered. Usually torsion occurs only on one side at a time. However, the same anatomic arrangement that allowed torsion to occur on the one side also exists on the other, and such a patient shoud have his good, remaining testicle fixed in position by a very simple surgical operation. Otherwise, at some time in the future he may lose that testicle as well.

Patients suffering from infertility because of a history of infection or torsion are generally sad cases where problems might have been avoided. For example, a patient from the West Coast two years ago underwent an episode of scrotal swelling on both sides which initially went untreated. By the time he saw a urologist who placed him on the appropriate antibiotic (resulting in rapid resolution of the epididymitis and swelling), he had already developed permanent obstruction.

Another patient had a more frightening but equally avoidable catastrophe. When he was fourteen his right testicle swelled up painfully and his doctor told him it was epididymitis, treated him with antibiotics, and did nothing else. Over the next three months the swollen testicle shrank to the size of a pea. He had lost his testicle from torsion. If anyone had taken the time to place a few stitches to fix the remaining left testicle in place to the scrotal skin so it would not twist, the disaster which occurred three years later would have been avoided. At that time, during a football game, his remaining left testicle suddenly twisted around, swelled up dramatically, and after three months this one also shrank, and he became a eunuch.

It was not until several years ago when he consulted a urologist that he realized that he had not had an infection, but rather torsion of the testicles. Torsion occurs unexpectedly only in people who are born with a testicle anatomically able to twist around within the scrotal sac. In most people the testicle is fixed in position so that it can't twist. In those whose testicles are twistable the problem is almost always found on both sides. Therefore the loss of one testicle is a warning to fix the other one before it is too late.

*General Illnesses.* Infections or generalized illnesses of almost any sort can have unexpected adverse effects on a man's fertility. Typical examples of common infections which reduce male fertility are general flu viruses, dental abscesses, recurrent acne, diarrhea, and any sort of general illness which can cause a fever. Any such disturbance frequently leads to a reduced production of sperm. I had performed a vasectomy reversal on a very nice doctor from the West Coast, and his sperm counts were normal within six months of the surgery. In fact he had over 100 million sperm per cc with good quality motility. Yet over the next year he failed to impregnate his wife and called me repeatedly asking why his sperm count had suddenly dropped to much lower levels of around fifteen million per cc with only 20 percent motility. He denied having any other illness or problem that could account for the decline in sperm production. Luckily he was due for a dental checkup, and his dentist discovered a substantial abscess behind several teeth which the patient had never really thought seriously about. However, he had been running fevers frequently over the last six months because of it. After the infection was cleared up by his dentist, his sperm count came back to 100 million sperm per cc with excellent motility. It is incredible that male infertility may be improved simply by sending the patient to a good dentist. Any infection can decrease sperm production.

Also there are a number of specific infections which attack the testicles or epididymis directly (rather than indirectly by elevating the temperature). Oddly enough, smallpox, a disease never seen in the United States anymore, was the commonest cause of azospermia (total absence of sperm in the ejaculate) in India. Almost 80 percent of men who come down with smallpox and survive have epididymal obstruction from the virus's direct attack on their epididymis. Tuberculosis also goes specifically to the epididymis to cause azospermia. Gonorrhea (which is on the increase in our society) can very easily result in obstruction of the epididymis or sperm duct if the antibiotic therapy is not instituted immediately. A more common problem in this country than gonorrhea, however, is the so-called "nonspecific epididymitis," which does not result from any obvious venereal disease, but behaves in the same fashion. The man may have had a nonspecific prostatitis preceding the epididymitis. Ordinary bacteria cultures usually reveal nothing. It is felt that these "nonspecific" infections are caused by unusual organisms that do not turn up on routine laboratory tests.

*Drugs.* A history of almost any medical problem requiring chronic drug therapy could be a culprit in the male's infertility. We recently saw a lawyer who had had no difficulty impregnating his wife several years before. They had a happy little four-year-old, but now had been trying unsuccessfully for two years to have a second child. He and his wife had seemed to be reasonably fertile, since she had become pregnant so quickly the first time they tried. Yet now his sperm count was terribly low with poor motility. He had a varicose vein of the testicle, which we were prepared to operate upon in an effort to improve his sperm count, but there was something in his history far more revealing. Two years before, just prior to the time they decided to try to have their second child, he had gone to his internist for a routine physical examination. Although he had no symptoms of any illness, the internist noted a few irregularities in his heartbeat on the electrocardiogram. He did not feel that these irregularities represented a grave risk to the patient, but after a complete and careful series of tests on his heart, decided it would be wise to place him on a drug called quinidine to control the abnormal heartbeats. It was right after starting this drug that his sperm count went down. The effects of most drugs on fertility have not yet been studied, and they should always be considered culprits, since anything that affects the body's normal functions can affect fertility.

*Hidden Testicles.* About one out of every two hundred male children is born with testicles that are in the abdomen rather than in the scrotum. These testicles are maintained at body temperature rather than at the cooler temperature of the scrotal sac. Unless operated on before five years of age, these children will usually have poor sperm-producing ability when they reach adulthood. Sometimes these cryptorchid (or hidden) testicles are so high up in the abdomen that the doctor cannot find them. He may then tell the parents that the child was born without testicles. Then, much to everyone's surprise, at age twelve or thirteen the child begins to undergo puberty. Actually the testicles were present, but so high up that the doctor could not locate them. The unfortunate thing about such an event is that although able to produce testosterone, these testicles will have lost forever their ability to produce sperm adequately, because they were not surgically brought down at an earlier age. Of course if only one testicle suffers from this problem, the patient will probably be fertile. In fact there are a great many men who have only one testicle and are perfectly fertile.

*Previous Surgery.* A history of surgery for hernia, hidden testicle, or hydrocoele of the testicle (common operations that are often performed in the patient's infancy or early childhood) can be a cause of later infertility. I received a letter last year from a doctor who did not identify himself or the patient about whom he was concerned. This doctor was a specialist in male fertility, and explained in a hand-scribbled note that, a few weeks before, he had operated on a fifteen-year-old boy because of a large varicose vein of the testicle that he thought was causing a lot of discomfort. The doctor confessed that a segment of the left vas deferens was removed accidentally during the operation. This unfortunate child had undergone a one-sided vasectomy at the age of fifteen without even realizing it. Fortunately his right testicle and vas deferens were spared, and he will probably remain fertile. All patients are not so lucky: sometimes the hernia or similar problem is on *both* sides, and sloppy surgery results in complete sterility.

*Diabetes.* Diabetes has a specific effect on male fertility that in most cases can be corrected, but which can be rather frightening at first to the patient. Since diabetic patients frequently undergo over the years a gradual degeneration of their "sympathetic" nerves which cause the bladder neck to close (and thereby force the ejaculate out of the penis), they may notice a gradual shrinkage of the volume of their ejaculate to the point where eventually they ejaculate nothing at all despite having a completely normal-feeling orgasm. Occasionally they may not even be aware of their problem until they are asked to produce a semen specimen for analysis. Actually they are ejaculating normal sperm, but it is going backward into their bladder rather than forward out the penis. By putting them on a simple pill that restimulates their weak "sympathetic" nerves, they can once again ejaculate forward and become fertile.

*Frequency of Sex.* A very important aspect of the history is the frequency and timing of intercourse. Certainly after prolonged periods of abstinence from ejaculation, the semen contains an abundant amount of sperm, but there are a high number which are dead or senescent. At the other extreme, daily ejaculation results in a lower sperm count, but the sperm are fresher. As simple as it seems, doctors still have not accurately decided whether it is better to have sex every day, or to wait until every other day, or every third day, to maximize the man's fertility potential. Certainly the sperm count may be better in a subfertile male who waits three days. Whether that single good count is more important than frequent ejaculation of poorer sperm counts is not certain. For example, a study in normal fertile men demonstrated the highest rate of pregnancy in couples who had intercourse every day. However, in men with lower sperm counts, this daily intercourse might not be so wise.

Techniques of intercourse are also relevant, and though not important in the very fertile couple, can cause problems when the man has a low sperm count. For example, if the wife is in the top position and the husband on the bottom, it would be very likely that a good deal of sperm would leak right out after intercourse. Also, if the wife gets up within a minute or so after ejaculation to go to the bathroom most of the sperm will leak out. Coital technique may not be very important in the average couple with high fertility, but in the couple with low fertility, small differences in sexual technique may help to maximize the chance for conception.

*Emotional Stress.* Emotional stress may possibly have an effect on sperm production. The findings on this issue are not yet clear. In 1933 a study was performed on prisoners sentenced to death who were kept waiting a long period before the moment of execution. Testicle biopsies were performed on these prisoners at various intervals prior to execution. Severe disturbances in sperm production and progressive deterioration of fertility were noted in many of them. Studies have also been performed on animals, designed to determine the effects of overcrowded conditions and repeated frustration. Such artificial social stress related to excessive population densities in rats has resulted in poor testicular function and diminished fertility. Young mice in overcrowded cages show inhibited and delayed puberty, and there is a decrease in the mother's average litter size. Similarly, when female mice in groups of ten to thirty are kept in small cages, their cycles become irregular and may stop altogether. Thus there are many studies in animals, and suggestive inferences in humans, which show that stress may play a role in male as well as female infertility.

*Past History of Fertility.* The most important aspect of a couple's medical history is whether they have ever been able to conceive together before, or whether perhaps in a previous marriage either the husband or the wife has been able to have children. When infertile couples are divorced, and each partner remarries, very often they have no difficulty getting pregnant. This is because infertility is usually due to relative deficiency in both partners rather than a major deficiency in one.

In most men who suffer from infertility problems, there will be no such revealing medical history. We only detail some of the things to watch out for to help the smaller number of patients in whom such events may have contributed to their low fertility. In most men with low sperm counts and poor fertility, we simply don't have any idea why they have their problem.

PHYSICAL EXAMINATION

Physical examination for male infertility is quite simple. The most important things to look for are the size of the testicles, and the presence of varicose veins in the scrotum.

*Size of the Testicles.* Since the tubules which make the sperm account for 98 percent of the testicle mass, a reduction in the sperm-producing cells will lead to a decrease in the testicle's size. But this is highly variable. Some men with large testicles are not fertile, and many men with small testicles are fertile. However, testicles less than one inch in diameter usually have some disturbance in sperm production.

If the testicle is small but the internal structure is normal, the patient may still be quite fertile. Often, however, a small testicle is a sign of deficient internal structure.

*Varicose Veins of the Testicles.* A varicose vein of the testicle, called a varicocele, is the most common treatable cause of male infertility. A varicose vein in the scrotum is caused by a leaky backflow valve in the vein leading from the testicle into the abdomen. When a man with this problem stands, blood from the abdomen drains down to engorge a dilated network of scrotal veins. These dilated varicose veins can be quite large when the man is standing. Yet when he lies down and feels his scrotal sac, the veins are no longer apparent. Ten percent of all men *normally* have a varicocele—and it does not appear to interfere with their fertility. Yet in infertile men, correction of the varicocele can lead to a dramatic improvement in the sperm count in 75 percent of cases. In fact, in men who have a varicocele, its surgical correction is the single most effective method of raising their sperm counts. How a varicocele affects sperm production is not really understood. There are many theories. Perhaps the most plausible is that warm blood from the abdomen is allowed to leak down into the scrotum whenever the patient is standing, and this throws the temperature-regulating mechanism of the scrotum out of kilter. The testicles are just too warm to work properly.

Just because the majority of men with varicoceles are perfectly fertile does not mean that men with this condition should take it too lightly. One and a half years ago I was going on a hike with my wife and children in one of our local parks. We happened to come across another couple, and though we had never met before, we got along quite well. I didn't see them again until five months later, when the husband called my office for a minor unrelated problem. In the course of a routine physical examination, I discovered an enormous varicocele in the left part of his scrotum. This didn't really seem to be bothering him, and it was not the reason he had come to me. I obtained a semen collection for analysis, not expecting to find any problem. He resisted at first, and I almost let him get out of it.

He and his wife wished to have children eventually, but certainly did not want them now. They had been married for ten years and she had been on birth control pills all that time. Furthermore, she intended to stay on the pills for several more years. The last thing on his mind was his fertility. Of course I expected to find a completely normal sperm count. What I found instead was only a rare sperm in the entire ejaculate. The few that I saw were dead. I explained to him the findings and he had a hard time believing it.

He and his wife decided that they still didn't want children for several more years, but they didn't like the idea of not being able to have them when they wanted them. We operated to correct the varicocele, and his sperm count, which had been close to zero, dramatically rose to higher levels over the course of the next six months. In the infertile man with a varicocele (as many as 20 percent to 30 percent of infertile men have a varicocele), surgical correction of this condition is more dramatically successful than any other therapy. Luckily most men with varicocele are fertile, but, for some unknown reason, in a small number of men varicocele is very harmful to sperm production.

## HORMONE STUDIES

There is still a lot of confusion about hormone testing and male infertility. In decades gone by, thyroid and adrenal tests would routinely be performed, and whether or not they were normal (they were virtually always normal), males were frequently put on thyroid supplements. With no great knowledge about thyroid function, many urologists would routinely put their patients on such therapy, hoping that in some sort of mystical hormonal fashion it would "pep them up" and improve their sperm count. I only mention this archaic approach because it is still practiced in many communities. Yet certainly all of the scientific studies on male infertility performed over the last ten years contraindicate this routine use of thyroid medication to try to stimulate sperm production, because it doesn't work. In fact, even patients with documented thyroid deficiencies who need to take medication because they truly have thyroid disease usually are fertile.

There are three hormones in the male that are very closely involved in sperm production. They are follicle-stimulating hormone (FSH), luteinizing hormone (LH), and testosterone. Until recently hormone tests were not widely available, but now almost any good laboratory in the country can measure these hormones in the blood. Blind reliance upon these tests, however, can be misleading.

Testosterone, the major male hormone produced by the testicle, has a concentration in blood which varies two- to threefold from hour to hour. The testicle changes so greatly its output of testosterone, with no apparent rhyme or reason, that it is very difficult to pinpoint if there is a deficiency in its production. It is only when the testosterone falls outside this wide range of variability that we would dare to call it abnormal. Thus a patient could indeed be suffering from a disease or defect in his testosterone production, and we would not be able to detect it simply by measuring it in the blood.

LH is the hormone released from the pituitary that stimulates the testicle to make testosterone. LH levels, like testosterone, vary dramatically from hour to hour. An elevation of LH above the normal range indicates either an inadequate number of Leydig cells (the cells in the testicle that make testosterone) or inadequate function of those Leydig cells. Very often a man with an elevated blood LH level, indicating poor testicle functioning, will have a normal testosterone level and normal male sex features. These are only normal, however, because of the overworking of his pituitary and brain, pouring out extra amounts of releasing hormone to make up for the deficiency in his testicles.

FSH is the most important of the three hormones for reflecting the testicle's sperm-producing capacity. When FSH is elevated, this generally reflects a specific defect in sperm production. Unfortunately, scientists do not really know exactly how FSH works to promote sperm production, and furthermore we do not know how testicular sperm production tells the brain to release less FSH. We simply know for a fact that if all of the sperm-producing cells of the testicle are absent, even though the rest of the testicle may be perfectly normal, the blood LH and testosterone remain normal, but the FSH goes up to high levels just as though the patient had been castrated.

## TESTICLE BIOPSY

At our present state of knowledge, if we really want to understand what is wrong with an infertile man's testicle, we simply have to resort in most cases to testicle biopsy. Testicle biopsy should rarely be performed on men whose sperm count is only in a moderately low range. However, it is very valuable for the more severe cases of male infertility. Unfortunately, often little information is derived from it because the technique for obtaining the biopsy in most hands is so poor that it becomes unreadable under the microscope. It will facilitate the husband's treatment only if performed and read by physicians who understand more than superficially how the testicle works.

A testicle biopsy involves taking a tissue sample through a one-quarter-inch incision in the scrotum. The procedure should take no more than five minutes, but it must be done expertly. Testicular tissue is so delicate that if the surgeon handles it in the way that he would handle most specimens removed for biopsy from other areas of the body, the microscopic architecture of the specimen would be so shattered as to make it very difficult to interpret. Furthermore, if the tissue is not properly excised, or is placed in formaldehyde (the usual fixative used for tissue specimens obtained from almost anywhere else in the body), it would become distorted beyond recognition. The tissue must be placed in a solution which is gentler. Most men consider their testicles rather dear to them, and though the testicle biopsy is quite harmless, a man should not have to part with a portion of one unless helpful information will be derived.

Contrary to expectation, the biopsy is not very painful. The patient should have minimal temporary discomfort, which is relieved simply by aspirin. It is like having a headache in the testicles for a few days.

After the specimen is fixed and stained, it is examined by the doctor under a microscope. If the specimen has been properly obtained, fixed, and stained, the doctor should be able to see before his own eyes a remarkable assembly line of sperm production. By looking at the various stages of sperm production along this assembly line, he will be able to tell whether there are an adequate number of precursors starting out at the beginning, whether there are weak spots along the production line, or whether there is a problem in the end stages of production when the sperm should be elongating and forming a tail.

What if the biopsy is completely normal? A testicle biopsy which appears normal usually indicates obstruction in the outflow system of the testes. Occasionally a normal testicle biopsy is a sign that a small testis is causing the low sperm count. In such a case the patient's pituitary hormones are probably elevated and driving the small testicle to work at greater than its expected capacity. Additional hormones administered to such patients can sometimes drive the testicles to produce even more sperm.

The worst finding on testicle biopsy is that there is a complete absence of any sperm or sperm-producing cells in the seminiferous tubules. The Leydig cells which make the male hormone, testosterone, are normal in these cases. There simply are no sperm of any kind. There is no possible treatment for a patient with this picture.

A third pattern found on testicle biopsy is maturation arrest. In this case sperm production may be proceeding properly in the early phases, but some missing catalyst is preventing further development of these spermatocytes into mature sperm. In different patients maturation arrest can occur at different phases of the sperm-production process, and presumably represent a different missing part in each case.

In men with the severest depression of sperm count, although all phases of the assembly line are generally deficient, it is the later stages that are most deficient. Thus the number of spermatozoa in the ejaculate reflects the later stages of sperm production most closely. We are now just beginning to understand what enzymes and what hormones influence the different stages of sperm production along the testicular assembly line. It is to be hoped that in the future a careful analysis of the testicle biopsy, particularly in men with maturation arrest, may help guide the appropriate therapy.

VASOGRAMS

When it is suspected that the sperm duct is obstructed, an X ray can be performed by injecting an opaque liquid. This test is called a vasogram. This X ray is not necessary (or advised) to diagnose obstruction. It should only be used as part of an operative procedure once the diagnosis of obstruction is made. The only two tests required to determine that there is obstruction to the outflow of sperm are a sperm count that reveals little or no sperm at all in the semen, and a normal testicle biopsy. In the presence of these two findings, obstruction will always be found somewhere, and a vasogram is not necessary to make that diagnosis. The vasogram is valuable but only as part of the total operative approach to correct obstruction to sperm outflow.

## Tests on the Female

Diagnosing the wife's role in a barren marriage may sometimes be more complicated than it need be. Going through expensive and sometimes painful tests without a clear understanding of what they are to accomplish is an intimidating experience which the woman is sometimes afraid to question. The female reproductive cycle is so intricate that she may even expect complicated and expensive testing. For most women, however, this should not actually be the case. We can correlate the complex series of hormonal events that regulate female fertility with a very simple series of observations that can be performed by most physicians in their office.

However, the usual pelvic examination performed yearly by the gynecologist along with a Pap smear tells little about fertility. I recently saw a couple who had been trying to have a baby for more than ten years. It was assumed that the wife was normal because whenever her gynecologist, a rather old and somewhat outdated fellow, performed a pelvic exam on her, he simply told her that she was a normal woman, patted her on the head, and told her not to worry. Women have been indoctrinated into thinking that if they have a normal pelvic exam and Pap smear once a year, their reproductive system is all right. Unfortunately this yearly pelvic exam does not tell why the wife isn't pregnant. On the other hand, expensive and complicated hormone tests are not always necessary either. The purpose of this section is to explain what tests are actually needed to evaluate fertility. A large number of tests are performed on women which often do not give any information that aids in treatment. Many tests are expensive and uncomfortable. Actually, the testing can be simple and inexpensive and yet give all the necessary information. Let's look at some of these tests and see what they really do and do not tell us.

HISTORY AND PHYSICAL

A normal menstrual history and a normal physical examination do not mean that a woman is fertile, but an abnormal history is a hint that there are problems. The clues to a woman's infertility may appear years before she has any interest in having children. When a girl's periods first begin at age twelve or thirteen, a stage in life known as menarche, they are naturally very irregular. However, by age fifteen or sixteen they should have stabilized so that they come about every twenty-eight days, are of four to five days' duration, and tend to be a bit heavier the first or the second day, tapering off to just a little spotting on the last day. There is a precise hormonal clockwork which regulates the development of the follicle, secretion of estrogen, buildup of a thick lining in the uterus prior to ovulation, the LH surge which induces ovulation, and conversion to a soft lining in the uterus after ovulation when the ruptured follicle starts making progesterone. If this intricately synchronized clockwork of hormonal events is out of tune, the periods may be irregular. In a fertile woman, the normal buildup of a firm, thick lining in the womb, followed by a lush softening of that lining in the second half of the month, leads to an even and neat flow of menstrual blood. The uterus has a fresh start with each new cycle. However, if there is no ovulation, the lining of the uterus builds up unevenly, and bleeding can occur irregularly.

When the number of days between menstrual periods varies too greatly, this is a sign of an error somewhere in the clockwork that regulates proper buildup of the lining of the womb, and is usually associated either with lack of ovulation or with poor ovulation. Certainly women with irregular periods can ovulate and get pregnant, but if they are ovulating, they are frequently ovulating late or they are not ovulating with each monthly cycle. Some women may ovulate only twice a year and have very mixed-up periods in between. If the husband has a very high sperm count, the woman may very well get pregnant the one time she does ovulate.

The only way of knowing clinically that a woman has ovulated is if she is producing progesterone in the second half of her cycle. Progesterone softens up the lining of the uterus so that a more complete and clean shedding of it will occur at the end of her cycle. When ovulation has not occurred, and progesterone has not been produced, the lining of the womb is somewhat tougher and flakes off in bits and pieces. Periods may not be painful or heavy until several months' worth of this inadequately shed lining has built up. Irregular periods indicate a step-by-step peeling off of the lining rather than a heavy shedding of its entire thickness.

Extremely painful periods may be a sign of a condition called endometriosis in which some of the tissue lining the inside of the womb is located in areas outside the womb. Thus when the lining of the womb begins to shed, similar shedding occurs outside the womb and causes pain. Not only is this an aggravating condition for the woman to endure, but such bleeding outside the womb can result in scarring and interference with the transport of the egg from the ovary to the tube.

Some women feel several hours of pain called *mittelschmerz* at the time of ovulation. This is a sharp, crampy sensation felt on one or the other side, depending on which ovary is extruding the egg. For reasons we don't understand, most women do not feel this pain. Those who do feel this pain can tell exactly when they are ovulating.

Using birth control pills will generally make irregular periods regular, because they artificially control the buildup and shedding of the lining of the womb. However, with the pill a much thinner lining develops and therefore the periods are much lighter. The woman who has had uncomfortable periods frequently is relieved of all of her menstrual discomfort when she goes on the pill.

Most women who do not ovulate regularly have a slightly increased amount of male hormone. It is not clear whether the increased production of male hormone is causing them not to ovulate, or whether their inability to ovulate is upsetting their hormonal clockwork to the point where too much male hormone is being produced. Regardless of which came first there is frequently a definite increase in male hormone output in women who are not ovulating regularly. For this reason it is important to check for subtle signs of increased male-hormone production. A small amount of hair on the breast, a slightly denser than usual amount of hair in the midline of the lower abdomen, a small amount of fuzzy hair around the anus, or even hair on the great toe are all signs of slightly elevated male hormone production.

Remember that the male makes female hormones, and the female makes male hormones. It is only the proportion of these hormones that determines how we function. A woman with elevated male hormones if anything may be more interested in sex than one with normal levels of male hormones. In the human a small amount of male hormone in the female does more to stimulate her sexual desire than do the female hormones.

Another sign of excess male hormone, which often turns up in the late teens and whose significance is not realized until ten or fifteen years later when a woman is unable to get pregnant, is acne. Very frequently acne which persists beyond the mid-teens in a girl is a sign of elevated male-hormone production associated with lack of ovulation. Oily skin has similar connotations. Thus menstrual irregularity, excessive pain, abnormal body hair distribution, oily skin, and acne can be clues to an ovulatory disturbance. However, to pinpoint the wife's ovulatory pattern accurately requires more than just guesswork.

AM I OVULATING?

*Basal Body Temperatures.* The most accurate and yet inexpensive method of determining ovulation is to keep a daily basal body temperature chart. The basal body temperature is the temperature immediately upon waking up in the morning, before getting out of bed or having any activity whatsoever. Before ovulation, this temperature will always be about one degree Fahrenheit lower than after ovulation. The production of progesterone (which can only occur after ovulation) raises the body's basal temperature one degree Fahrenheit and it is this event that we are measuring. Charts for recording these monthly temperatures are available at almost any pharmacy, or from your doctor (see Graph 1). Any thermometer will do, but it may be easier to read the temperature with a special Ovulindex thermometer (again, available at any pharmacy).

The only pitfall with this otherwise superb and inexpensive way of determining your ovulation is that if the temperatures are not taken first thing in the morning, before you even move to get out of bed, they may give a falsely elevated reading and be difficult to interpret. Every evening before going to bed you must place the thermometer by your nightstand within easy reach. If you forget to do this, you will have to get out of bed in the morning to get to your thermometer. Even this slight degree of activity can raise your temperature above the basal level and make that day's temperature reading worthless. Upon awaking in the morning you simply grasp the thermometer before doing anything else, put it in your mouth under the tongue for three minutes, and lie still.

When you have taken your temperature, you then record it on a chart according to the date and the day of the cycle. The day on which menstrual bleeding begins, even if only lightly, is considered

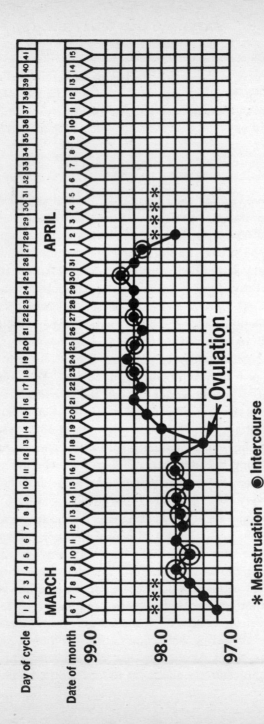

Graph 1. Normal Basal Body Temperature (BBT).

day one of the menstrual cycle. During menstruation mark your temperature with an X, and when menstruation is completed use a circle. On the top line of the chart record the day of the cycle (one through twenty-eight or higher), and on the bottom line put the date. At the end of the cycle, when the first day of the next menstruation begins, mark an X instead of a circle; then go to the next section, and begin charting your temperature for another month. After you have finished taking and recording your temperature in the morning, you can go about your daily activities. In the evening make sure that before you go to sleep, you shake down your thermometer and put it on your nightstand within easy reach for the next morning.

Remember that the temperature can be affected by such things as colds, flu viruses, keeping late hours, or having a poor night's sleep. Make sure to note such events on the chart so that if there are a few atypical readings that don't go along with the rest of the temperature pattern, you will be able to discount them. Remember the basal body temperature refers to the body temperature after a night of a normal, restful sleep. The body temperature normally reaches its lowest levels after all mental and muscular activity has ceased for several hours. That is why the best time to record this basal temperature is just upon awakening. Your temperature during the rest of the day is affected by your daily activities and will not be an accurate reflection of whether you are making progesterone, and consequently whether or not you have ovulated.

The basal body temperature of a fertile woman follows a very characteristic pattern during each menstrual cycle. A low temperature range spans the first fourteen days beginning from the first day of menstruation. This low range is generally in the area of 97.2° F to 97.6° F. Around day fourteen there is a sudden increase in the basal body temperature (up to one degree) which is maintained daily until menstruation begins and the temperature drops again. If instead of menstruating you become pregnant, the temperature will remain elevated, as it was in the second half of the cycle, because progesterone continues to be produced. This temperature phenomenon is dependent on the hormones your body produces. Progesterone, which is only produced *after* ovulation, is what increases your basal body temperature. If pregnancy occurs, the production of progesterone continues and the temperature remains elevated in contrast to the abrupt drop that occurs with menstruation (see Graph 2). If the temperature does not go up, you have not ovulated (see Graph 3). If the temperature goes up after day seventeen or eighteen in the cycle, rather than on day fourteen or fifteen, this indicates delayed ovulation. If menstruation occurs less than twelve days after the rise in temperature, this indicates a condition called short luteal phase (see Graph 4). Both delayed ovulation and a short luteal phase can prevent conception as readily as the lack of ovulation. In fact delayed ovulation, as indicated by a late rise in temperature, may even indicate a false ovulation; that is, your follicle is simply beginning to make progesterone even though an egg may not have been extruded. Keep in mind always that we have no way of telling directly whether or not you have ovulated. All of our methods of measurement are indirect, based upon progesterone production.

Of all the expensive and complicated methods for determining ovulation, there is none as effective and accurate as this simple and inexpensive temperature chart. Frequently this chart is misinterpreted, however, and the patient thinks that she should wait until the temperature goes up (indicating ovulation) before having intercourse. Actually the temperature does not go up until one day after ovulation and by that time the egg is no longer capable of being fertilized, the cervix is closed, and the cervical mucus has become hostile to sperm. Thus, waiting for the temperature to rise before having intercourse is not a way of maximizing the chances of conception but is rather an excellent method of rhythm birth control. Intercourse should take place one or two days prior to the temperature rise.

*Examination of the Cervical Mucus During the Monthly Cycle.* Although the basal body temperature chart is the best single method of determining when ovulation occurs, it should be double-checked

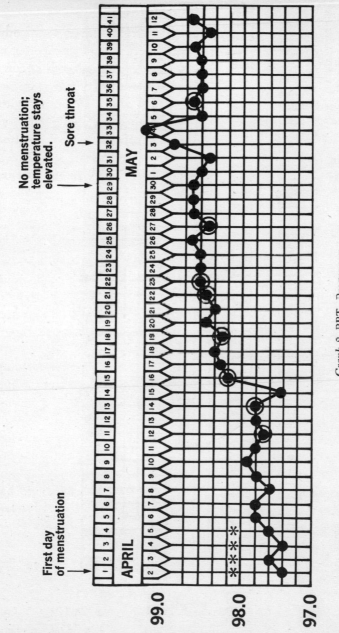

Graph 2. BBT—Pregnancy.

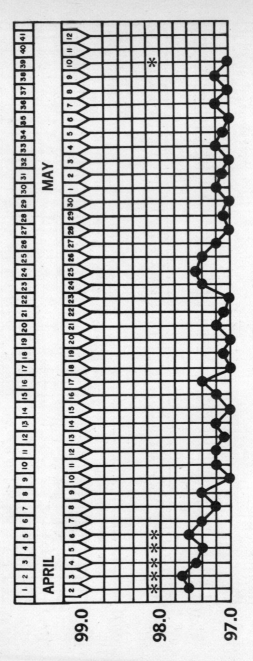

Graph 3. BBT—Anovulation.

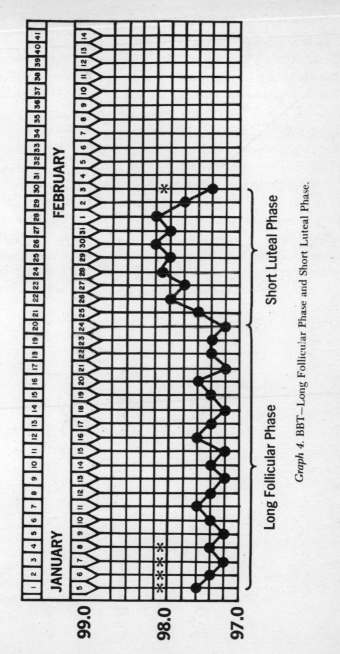

Graph 4. BBT—Long Follicular Phase and Short Luteal Phase.

with another extremely simple method, the examination of the cervical mucus on various days of the cycle (see Fig. 11). During the earliest phase of the cycle, the cervix is closed and very little cervical mucus is produced (Fig. 12). However, beginning around day nine or ten, under the influence of estrogen produced by the developing follicle, the production of cervical mucus begins to increase and the cervix begins to open slightly. When follicular production of estrogen has reached its maximum, usually around day thirteen or fourteen in a normal cycle, the cervix is gaping open and one can actually see into it because of the optically clear, copious, watery cervical mucus flowing out. At this time, one or two days prior to ovulation, the cervical mucus is most receptive to invasion by sperm and the cervix is wide open in anticipation of their entrance (Fig. 13). The physician can actually grasp a sample of this cervical mucus with a small clamp, and spread it out several

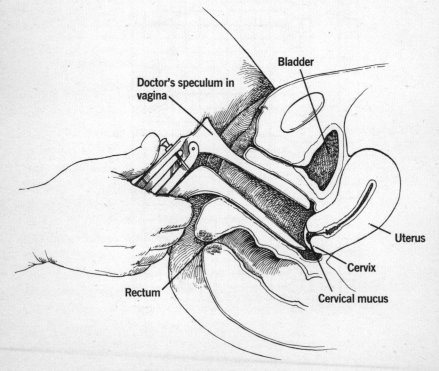

*Figure 11.* Pelvic Examination.

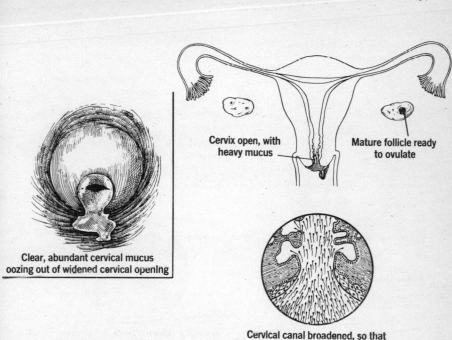

Clear, abundant cervical mucus oozing out of widened cervical opening

Cervix open, with heavy mucus

Mature follicle ready to ovulate

Cervical canal broadened, so that sperm invade cervical mucus easily

*Figure 12.* Just Before Ovulation.

inches. It will not break. It has the perfect, clear, copious, elastic consistency required for the sperm to launch a successful invasion.

Then when the woman ovulates, and progesterone is produced, the entrance to the cervix will dramatically close and the production of cervical mucus will come almost to a standstill. What mucus is left will be sticky and tacky and will have lost its optical clarity. At this point sperm would have no chance of invading the mucus. If the physician sees a so-called "preovulatory" cervix (with a gaping opening and optically clear, abundant mucus) on day fourteen, if the temperature goes up the next morning, and if the cervical opening then closes abruptly, he can be fairly certain the woman is ovulating properly. If, however, her temperature never rises and the cervical opening never closes until after menstruation, this indicates that she is not ovulating.

Just because a woman ovulates properly in one month does not

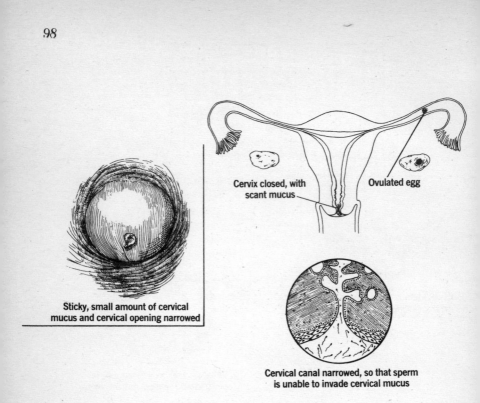

Cervix closed, with scant mucus

Ovulated egg

Sticky, small amount of cervical mucus and cervical opening narrowed

Cervical canal narrowed, so that sperm is unable to invade cervical mucus

*Figure 13.* After Ovulation.

mean she will do so in another month. Many women will ovulate only every other cycle or every third cycle. This reduces their chance of becoming pregnant, especially if the husband's semen analysis is borderline. If the cervical opening is gaping with abundant mucus on day twenty, but then the temperature goes up on day twenty-one and the cervical opening closes, then ovulation is occurring late in the cycle (see Graph 5). This also results in a lesser likelihood of conception. If the temperature goes up on day fifteen (corroborated by simultaneous closing of the cervical opening, with a reduction in cervical mucus production), but menstruation begins eight days after this rise in temperature, this is what is called a short luteal phase. The corpus luteum is not producing progesterone for long enough to support the lining of the uterus. This also results in diminished likelihood of conception.

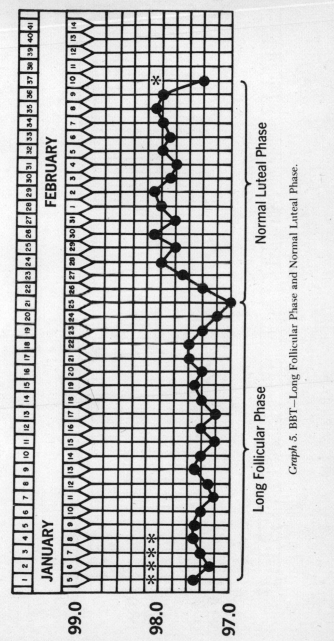

*Graph 5.* BBT—Long Follicular Phase and Normal Luteal Phase.

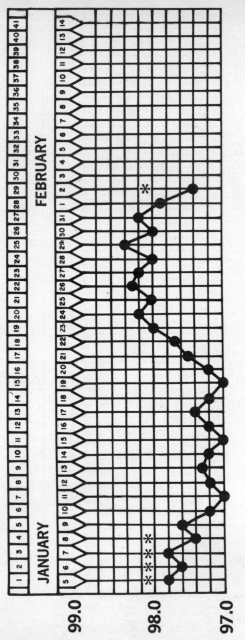

Graph 6. BBT—Slow Rise of Temperature at Ovulation.

100

Occasionally one sees the temperature begin to rise slowly but not reach its proper "luteal" level until about four days later (see Graph 6). This patient may or may not be ovulating; but remember that we never really know for sure whether she is ovulating, only that she is making progesterone. Slow rises in temperature associated with a gradual rather than a dramatic closing of the cervical opening may also indicate a decreased likelihood of conception. Occasionally the temperature may appear to rise, indicating ovulation, but the cervical opening does not close at the same time. The cervical opening may continue to appear gaping with abundant and copious mucus for several days after the temperature has supposedly risen. This is the reason that the physician must double-check the cervix against the basal body temperature charts. If they don't match, there may be a problem. Evaluating the female this way usually takes about three cycles to determine whether there is an ovulatory problem or not.

I am not suggesting reliance upon simple and inexpensive tests for ovulation because of any lack of respect for the sophisticated complexity of hormonal events taking place in the proper ovulatory cycle. However, the only other way to obtain this kind of daily information is to do blood hormone tests every day during two cycles, which tends to be extremely expensive. Obtaining blood hormone tests on only one or two days during the month would give very little information. If progesterone is positive in the latter half of the cycle, we can say that at some time or other the follicle has ruptured and perhaps ovulation has taken place. That is all we can say. Unless we test for blood levels of FSH, LH, estrogen, and progesterone every day for two cycles, we cannot possibly gain as much information about ovulation as we can by simply taking the temperature and watching the cervix.

## BLOOD HORMONE TESTS

To do an adequate hormone evaluation of the female would require almost daily blood tests because of the changing hormone levels with each day of the cycle. Such an approach, however, is expensive and impractical. Thus most fertility specialists rely heavily on the indirect indications of hormone balance just described. The only occasion on which hormones really need to be monitored daily is in the woman whose ovulation must be induced by a very powerful drug called Pergonal. Under these circumstances the estrogen levels in the blood must be checked every day in order to determine the proper dose. Otherwise a complicated battery of hormone tests is rarely needed.

Yet, to understand the hormonal events which the basal body temperature measures, we will review what the hormones would show if we were indeed to test them daily. The key hormones are FSH and LH released by the pituitary gland, and estrogen and progesterone released by the ovary, along with a smaller proportion of testosterone and other male hormones. The chart on page 28 in Chapter 1 summarizes what all of these hormones are doing during the month to stimulate and inhibit each other. On day one of menstruation, FSH goes up, and stimulates the follicle to produce estrogen. As estrogen is produced by the follicle, it depresses the pituitary's production of FSH. Thus during the first two weeks of the cycle, as the estrogen level goes up, the FSH level goes down. The rising estrogen begins to crescendo by day twelve and stimulates the pituitary gland to release a huge and sudden burst of the hormone LH. This sudden burst of LH by the pituitary causes ovulation. The ruptured follicle then becomes the corpus luteum, and begins to manufacture progesterone after ovulation. In the ideal twenty-eight-day cycle, this crescendo of events occurs at about day fourteen.

During the first two weeks of the cycle, the only female hormone produced by the ovary is estrogen. During the second two weeks of the cycle (assuming ovulation has taken place), the ovary produces mostly progesterone and some estrogen. The addition of progesterone converts the lining of the uterus from a relatively thick, hard, "proliferative" surface to a more soft, spongy "secretory" surface.

The corpus luteum (the ruptured follicle which makes the hormone progesterone) normally has a life span of about fourteen days. The only thing that can prolong its function is a pregnancy. In the absence of a pregnancy, the corpus luteum rather dramatically ceases to make hormones. When the hormone levels drop to near zero, the lining of the uterus is shed. This is the first day of menstruation. Because menstruation reflects a reduction of hormone production by the ovaries to near zero, the FSH level jumps abruptly to high levels and the cycle begins once again.

It is impossible to say on any particular day what is a "normal" level for any of these hormones, because the normal level varies from day to day according to the intricate clockwork of the monthly period. Luckily, estrogen and progesterone both have very obvious effects on the basal body temperature, the cervix, and the cervical mucus, which can be used as less expensive indicators of the woman's cyclic hormone balance.

The initial rise of FSH on day one is essential. Without this initial rise in FSH to stimulate follicle development, none of the other events of the cycle will occur in proper sequence. Although ovulation is actually triggered by a rapid rise in the circulating levels of estrogen on days twelve to fourteen, causing the pituitary to release LH, the initial condition required for a normal cycle is a high level of FSH during menstruation.

If the primitive region of the brain, the hypothalamus, is not functioning properly, this complicated cycling mechanism will not work and the woman will not ovulate. This may be one reason why stress, anxiety, worry, and lack of sleep can prevent ovulation. Unless the hypothalamus is properly tuned and not burdened by anxiety, ovulation may be disturbed.

It is usually impossible to determine precisely why a woman is not ovulating. The normal ovulatory function of the menstrual system relies on a very complicated and dynamic coordination of interrelating hormonal events. Whatever the cause of poor ovulation, the hormonal picture in almost all cases is a low FSH level at the beginning of the cycle, a failure of the brain to respond to rising estrogen levels at mid-cycle, and too much male hormone.

Lack of ovulation is a true disease and should not be regarded simply as a problem with becoming pregant. Even if the woman does not want to become pregnant, the hormonal imbalance resulting from or causing poor ovulation leads to heavy buildup of a hard uterine lining that does not shed properly like the soft lining of an ovulatory woman. Not only can this lead to irregular bleeding and occasionally a painful ovarian enlargement (which may even necessitate surgery), but over many years it can lead to the development of cancer of the lining of the womb. So the problem of not getting pregnant because of poor ovulation may be far greater than simply the barrenness of the marriage.

## ENDOMETRIAL BIOPSY

After ovulation has occurred, the lining of the uterus becomes soft, and under the influence of progesterone forms what is called a secretory endometrium. If ovulation has not occurred, then in the second half of the cycle, instead of a soft, spongy, secretory lining, there will be a hard proliferative lining, indicating that no progesterone has been produced. One way of testing to see if a woman has ovulated is, in the second half of the cycle, to examine under the microscope a tiny piece of that lining. This is called an endometrial biopsy. The procedure is actually quite simple, and can be performed in almost any gynecologist's office. This test only involves a brief, wincing moment of pain and it is very commonly done nowadays as part of the evaluation for ovulation. This procedure cannot give quite the same information about daily events of the woman's cycle as that which can be obtained from the basal body temperature and observation of the cervix, but it is helpful.

I saw a patient recently who had been scheduled for an endometrial biopsy to be performed by her gynecologist in two weeks, just before the time she was expected to menstruate. On day twelve, her cervix was wide open and releasing a good amount of clear cervical mucus. On day sixteen, her cervix was completely closed, and there was no mucus at all. At the same time her basal body temperature showed a prompt rise. She asked whether I really thought she needed this endometrial biopsy in view of the fact that her basal body temperatures and her two pelvic examinations indicated that she had ovulated properly around day fifteen. I was embarrassed to realize that she was right. We had all the information we needed with these simple, relatively painless, and very inexpensive tests.

It is never a bad idea to question your physican tactfully about what he is doing and why he is doing it. If you have a sufficient understanding of what he is trying to accomplish, you may become his best consultant. If he is unable to discuss his diagnostic and therapeutic decisions rationally, then you may have to look else-where for someone with whom you are more compatible. Certainly, I learned a lot from this patient; I was reflexively intending to allow her to go through an extra test that would give us no new useful information in helping her conceive. I didn't find out until four weeks later that at the time she was already pregnant. Had we performed the unnecessary test, the pregnancy might have been lost.

## X RAYS OF THE UTERUS AND TUBES

Thus far we have dwelt only on the most important aspect of female infertility, the ovulatory menstrual cycle. However, in many cases the tubes that carry the egg to the site of fertilization may be blocked or restricted in their movement. Thus, failure to conceive might be due to purely physical factors, even though ovulation may occur normally. The most obvious case in point is the woman who has had her tubes tied; that is, she has undergone sterilization. However, many women have blockage of the tubes because of previous infections, and sometimes these are infections they never even knew they had. Even a simple case of appendicitis in youth could result in scarring around the area of the tubes which could interfere with pickup of the egg from the ovary. One of the easiest ways to determine whether the tubes are structurally intact is through an X ray called a hysterosalpingogram, which is slightly painful, but which does not require hospitalization. The woman is given a pelvic examination, and a liquid which is opaque to X rays is injected through her cervix. An X ray is then taken, and the doctor can see a beautiful outline of the cavity of the uterus as well as the tubes (Fig. 14). If the tubes are open without obstruction, this liquid should spill freely into the abdominal cavity, and this is readily seen when the X ray is taken.

Occasionally, however, the X ray may give an impression that

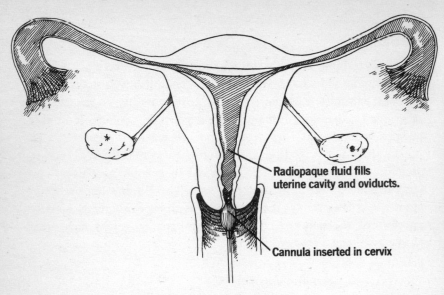

Radiopaque fluid fills
uterine cavity and oviducts.

Cannula inserted in cervix

*Figure 14.* Hysterosalpingogram.

the tubes are blocked when they really are not. Remember that the tiny canal that connects the uterus to the tubes has a valve which slows down the sperm trying to get into the tube. Consequently the X-ray contrast fluid sometimes may not go beyond the uterus simply because of spasms in the valve.

It is not sufficient simply to determine that the tubes are open. The fluid must spill freely into the abdominal cavity without accumulating in pockets. Pockets of fluid would indicate scarring outside the tube which can restrict its tentaclelike grasping of the egg. X ray does not always show this kind of scarring. The tube is not simply an alley through which the egg must roll like a bowling ball to reach the womb. The tube is a magnificently complicated structure which must have complete freedom of movement in order to ensure that the properly prepared egg is not just wasted in the abdominal cavity.

Performing this test accurately requires gentleness on the part of the gynecologist, and a full explanation of what is happening. Otherwise, the patient's anxiety itself may interfere with the performance of an adequate X ray. We recently saw a patient who was referred for blocked tubes. However, two months after we saw her, she became pregnant, indicating that earlier X rays—which seemed to indicate blockage—were in error.

## LAPAROSCOPY

Much information can be obtained about the tubes by actually looking inside the abdomen with a telescope inserted through the belly button (Fig. 15). This telescope, called a laparoscope, was designed specifically to allow a very detailed examination of the inside of the abdomen. The uterus, tubes, and ovaries can be freely inspected without the necessity of making a large exploratory incision. This procedure generally has to be performed with the patient anesthetized, and therefore may require a day in the hospital. Some gynecologists perform this procedure under local anesthesia, but most use general anesthesia. Laparoscopy is usually performed by the gynecologist who would eventually be performing tubal surgery if any obstruction or scarring is found.

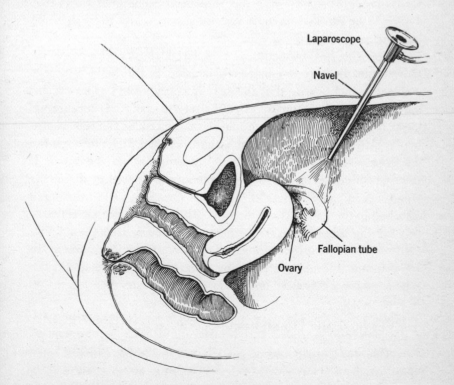

*Figure 15.* Laparoscopy.

Laparoscopy can reveal adhesions from previous infection that may be blocking the tubes, as well as more subtle adhesions outside the tube that could interfere with their ability to pick up the egg. Laparoscopy can allow one to examine the surface of the ovaries to see if there is a bubblelike or scarred appearance which suggests that ovulation is not occurring. Furthermore, laparoscopy is the only way of making a firm diagnosis of endometriosis. Endometriosis is an accumulation of the normal lining tissue of the uterus in areas outside the uterus. Such endometrial implants are a major cause of infertility. If there is any doubt as to the results of an X ray, laparoscopy can also be used as a confirmatory procedure by injecting a blue-colored liquid into the uterus through the cervix, and observing through the telescope whether this fluid spills freely through the tube into the abdomen. Sometimes tubes that appear to be blocked on an X ray are shown really to be open on laparoscopy.

After this full inspection is completed, the laparoscope is removed and the tiny one-half-inch incision in the belly button is stitched in such a way that the scar is rarely visible. The patient only has a minimum amount of pain after the operation because the incision is so tiny. She goes home the same day or the next morning. A skilled laparoscopist can actually correct, right through the telescope, some of the milder tubal problems that may be found. If there are filmy adhesions without blood vessels within them, the laparoscopist can cut right through them using a little instrument attached to the end of the telescope. This may be all that is necessary for the tubes to be sufficiently mobilized so that their tentaclelike action can grasp the egg effectively. If denser adhesions or more formidable obstructions are found, however, the patient is scheduled for a definitive operation at a later date.

### THE CERVICAL MUCUS AND IMMUNOLOGICAL TESTING

There is a great deal of speculation that some cases of infertility may be due to the wife's development of an immune reaction to the husband's sperm. We live in a hostile world surrounded by an infinite swarm of bacteria, viruses, parasites, and microscopic creatures of the most hideous varieties which would like nothing more than to feast upon us. Our constant protection against the eternal threat of invasion by these infectious organisms is our immune system. Any living thing which our body recognizes as foreign to our own tissue stimulates the production of antibodies which specifically attack that invading organism and kill it. Our white blood cells then move into the area to dispose of the dead carcasses of bacteria and viruses that have tried unsuccessfully to get in. Frequently bacteria and viruses do get a temporary foothold (such as the flu, a cold, or even a case of pneumonia), but it takes very little time for our immune systems to overwhelm them. Occasionally we need a little help from antibiotics, but without the help of that remarkable antibody system designed to overcome any foreign invader, no antibiotic medication would be of any use.

Occasionally the immune system may produce adverse rather than beneficial effects. If the patient has a kidney transplant, our immune system recognizes the foreign kidney as an enemy, and attacks it. Why then shouldn't the female uterus think of invading sperm as enemies and set up a similar immune response? Actually, one could go a step further and ask why the baby growing within the womb is not also thought of as foreign, and similarly destroyed by the mother's antibodies. This is clearly an area of much speculation, and most of the scientific studies in it have been contradictory. Somehow the body has a remarkable, and as yet totally inscrutable, mechanism for recognizing that the new baby living within the mother's womb is not to be rejected or attacked by antibodies. The same protection appears to be conferred upon the sperm so that they don't stimulate an antibody response with each episode of intercourse.

Although sperm antibodies are found in infertile women, they are also found in women of proven fertility. The thought that a wife is "allergic," or immune, to her husband's sperm can be staggering. Most of our methods of detecting these sperm antibodies are crude. Furthermore, the mere presence of antibodies to sperm in the blood in no way means that the invasion of sperm can be stopped by them. If sperm antibodies are ever to affect the woman's fertility, it is thought that they would have to get into the cervical mucus and attack the sperm cells there.

However, a simpler and more reliable test than measuring sperm antibodies in the blood is to check the cervical mucus for sperm penetration. If the wife's cervical mucus shows good survival of her husband's sperm, then sperm antibody tests need not be considered.

The most common cause of a finding of poor sperm penetration into the cervical mucus when the man's semen analysis is normal is that the test was performed at the wrong time of the woman's cycle. Usually it is simply a matter of having obtained the postintercourse cervical mucus on the wrong day, and rarely implies an immunological problem. In fact the usual solution to a truly "hostile" cervical mucus (verified by the sperm penetration test) is simply to give the wife a little estrogen supplement on days ten through fourteen of her cycle. This usually (but not always) solves problems associated with "hostility" of the mucus.

### Summary

The fact that a woman is not yet pregnant may simply be a mathematical inevitability, and patience may be the only treatment required. Although the series of events in both man and woman leading to conception is extraordinarily beautiful and intricate, the actual testing required if you have not yet conceived is relatively simple and inexpensive. On the other hand, these tests must be performed correctly. Neither you nor your doctor should be deceived into thinking that a normal pelvic exam performed once a year with a Pap smear is adequate to assure that a woman is fertile. Furthermore, a single sperm count performed on a specimen brought in a condom six hours after intercourse is inadequate for telling a woman that her husband is infertile. Answering the question "Why aren't we pregnant?" requires a simple but disciplined and systematic approach.

# ·4·

# Treatment of the Female

## What Anxiety Can Do to Fertility

One of the most remarkable patients of the famous fertility authority from Belgium, Dr. Robert Schoysman, was a beautiful thirty-year-old woman who felt that the future of her marriage depended gravely upon getting pregnant. She felt a medieval obligation to provide her husband with a son, feeling that otherwise she would have failed as a wife. After a year and a half, when she was still not pregnant, she consulted with all the leading authorities in Europe, and finally saw Dr. Schoysman. Her periods were irregular and frequently delayed several weeks, so that, very often, she would think that she was pregnant, only to be disillusioned by the arrival of her period several weeks later. Finally she developed a very rare condition called false pregnancy, in which her periods stopped altogether and she developed outward symptoms of pregnancy. She reported to the clinic month after month, insisting that she was pregnant, but her pregnancy tests were consistently negative.

False pregnancy is a rare but very real condition in which a woman so intensely wants to be pregnant that her abdomen actually expands, her periods stop, and she appears to any casual observer to be pregnant. When one such woman came to the obstetrics clinic, the doctors examined her very carefully, and obtained pregnancy tests which each time came back negative. Each time they told her she was not pregnant, she calmly informed them that they were mistaken. Nine months came and she looked as though she was just about ready to deliver a baby, but careful examination showed no fetal heartbeat, and pregnancy tests were still negative. All of her abdominal enlargement was simply body contour and fatty growth which develops in this rare condition. However, thirteen months after she first developed the false pregnancy, her pregnancy test suddenly became positive. Several months later, good fetal heart sounds could be heard.

This woman's false belief that she was pregnant relieved her anxiety so that she was finally able to ovulate normally and become pregnant. This case underscores the mysterious and profound effect which the primitive region of the brain, the hypothalamus, can have upon fertility.

The examples of couples who solved their infertility problems simply by allaying anxiety are countless. One couple had been trying for three years to have children, with no success. They were both thirty-five years old and were finally beginning to feel that their situation was hopeless. They had received a variety of conflicting opinions from different physicians. None of their physicians gave them a very comfortable or relaxed feeling. The husband was told that he had a very low sperm count. The wife was told that she was ovulating, because her periods were regular. When I examined him, he had a sperm count of twenty-two million sperm per cc, with 90 percent motility of excellent Grade III and Grade IV quality. I first saw her on day twenty-three of her monthly cycle, and explained to her that the opening of her cervix was closed, which indicated that she did ovulate, but that I would need to examine her regularly over the next two months, to determine just when she ovulated and what the quality of her ovulation was. I assured them that her husband's sperm count was quite sufficient to impregnate her and encouraged them to enjoy intercourse on a regular basis, and not to worry about timing. After she menstruated, I examined her regularly during her next cycle and saw the cervix opening properly on day ten and secreting excellent clear mucus, which became maximum on day fifteen. Her temperature went up on day sixteen and when I examined her then, her cervix was closed tightly, and I told her that she had ovulated right on schedule.

As I was scratching my head some time later, trying to figure out what might account for the fact that she had not gotten pregnant in three years, I got an excited telephone call that she had just received word from her gynecologist that she was pregnant, and couldn't thank me enough. *I had not done anything,* except systematically examine both her and her husband, and convey to them the secure feeling that we were going to attack their problem logically. I have seen countless cases like this one. Indeed, about 20 percent of couples with infertility achieve pregnancy before the doctor has a chance to initiate any treatment.

## Timing of Intercourse, Position, and Techniques

Most people who complain of infertility have simple problems such as infrequency of sex at the appropriate time in the cycle or poor positioning during sex– often associated by chance with marginal sperm counts and irregular ovulation. Simply improving the timing and techniques of intercourse may be sufficient to allow pregnancy, without fancy medical intervention and therapy. Animals always know just when to time their intercourse, because their periodic rise in estrogen, just prior to ovulation, is what induces them to desire intercourse. They have sex only during this obvious period when ovulation is imminent and pregnancy is most likely to occur. Humans are interested in sex at almost any time of the month, and we cannot be assured of the dull but proper timing that all other animals who are trying to raise a family enjoy.

The method of ejaculation in many animals is also less wasteful than in humans. Pigs, for example, ejaculate a full pint of semen into their sow, during an incredibly long orgasm. To make sure that none of this enormous volume of sperm leaks back out, the pig has grooves at the end of his penis which match the grooves in the cervix of the sow. The boar thus literally screws his penis into her cervix, obtaining a tight lock prior to ejaculation. Through a somewhat different mechanism, dogs also become tightly locked in the vagina of their female partner during intercourse, and the ejaculate cannot leak out. Humans do not have such well-designed mechanisms of timing or technique. Although we are very highly developed creatures, our reproductive apparatus is simply not as efficient as it might be, and improving the timing and technique of intercourse may, in couples with otherwise marginal fertility, be a simple solution to their problem.

A thirty-six-year-old man was recently referred to me for a low sperm count which supposedly caused his marriage to be barren. He and his thirty-six-year-old wife had been trying for the last five years to have a baby, without success. She had had very careful gynecological evaluations, which showed regular ovulation, no blockage in her tubes, and no endometriosis. In short, a very thorough evaluation had turned up nothing in her, and the blame for their infertility was placed on her husband's sperm count of twenty-two million sperm per cc. When I examined his semen, however, the quality was superb. He had 90 percent motility, almost all Grade III and Grade IV, with superb forward progression. The couple was having regular intercourse, at least every two or three days. Their sex life was active, vigorous, and frequent enough to have easily allowed impregnation during the fertile time of her cycles. The only unusual aspect of their intercourse was that she was in the habit of getting up within a minute of ejaculation, and going to the bathroom. There was thus considerable leakage of his semen out of her vagina. They had not stopped to think that this might be a problem. If his sperm count were higher, this habit of theirs would probably not have made any difference. I asked her to stay lying down for a full half hour after ejaculation, and only then get up to go to the bathroom. Two months later she called up, full of excitement, to tell me that after five years of trying to conceive, and going through several thousands of dollars' worth of testing, she was finally pregnant.

There are all kinds of positions in which couples may prefer to copulate, and these preferences may vary from month to month. In fact, modern sex books and magazine articles boast of all the different types of positions and contortions that the sexually active couple can utilize to increase their gratification. For the average couple all of these different positions will not have any effect on fertility, but a couple with a marginal sperm count just cannot afford to lose any sperm by leakage out of the vagina. The position of intercourse that allows the greatest contact of the semen with the cervical mucus is the simple traditional approach with the woman on the bottom and the man on the top. It also helps a little to have a pillow underneath the woman's bottom, so as to raise her vagina at a slight angle to help prevent semen from leaking out of the vagina after ejaculation. One only need stay in this position for thirty minutes after ejaculation, because any sperm that have not gained access to the cervical mucus within a half hour will not be able to do so later. They will be quite tired out by that burst of activity which is conferred upon them at the moment of ejaculation, and without the nourishing help of the cervical mucus protecting them from the acidity of the vagina, the sperm remaining after a half hour weaken and die. Thus any semen that leaks out after a half hour is of no consequence.

Perhaps even more important than the position of intercourse is the frequency and timing of intercourse. Many couples are so anxious about having intercourse at exactly the right time that they may abstain for a whole week just prior to the day or evening when the wife thinks she should be ovulating. The doctor is usually the culprit in this overrigorous scheduling of sex, and the wife may feel that they must abstain until the gynecologist gives her the go-ahead. This kind of overattention to regulating the precise night during which intercourse will be allowed can create so much anxiety that often ovulation does not take place anyway.

An acquaintance of mine, who I did not realize was having fertility problems, came into my office somewhat frantic one day, and begged that I see him as a patient. He simply couldn't take the strain anymore, and was hoping there was something I could do to help. He and his wife had been trying to have children for a year. Six months earlier she had consulted with her gynecologist. He had her take her basal body temperatures, which was fine, but he told her to abstain from intercourse for five days before her temperature went up, and only then to have sex. Her cycles had never been terribly regular, but when she was given this directive they became totally unpredictable, lasting twenty days one month and forty-five days another time. Her basal body temperature charts were difficult to interpret, but the couple tried to read into each little temperature elevation the possibility that she was about to ovulate. They did not realize that what the chart was truly showing was that she had stopped ovulating altogether. Sometimes, instead of abstaining for five days, they would abstain for as long as a week and a half, because her periods were becoming so irregular that she had no idea what was happening, but she was still trying in some way to pinpoint ovulation. Her original overanxiety about not conceiving during the first six months coupled with the rigidity of their sex life during the next six months (not to mention its infrequency) was about to lead to a divorce.

I saw both of them together, and explained the basal body temperature charts once again, pointing out that they should in no way gear their sex schedule to that chart. I was only interested in obtaining the temperatures so we could determine whether she was ovulating and how well she was ovulating. I advised them simply to have sex whenever they wanted. His sperm count showed ninety-five million sperm per cc, with 85 percent motility and excellent forward progression of sperm. With her history of irregular periods, I assumed we would find some ovulatory disturbance. Much to my surprise, her first month's basal body temperature chart showed a prompt ovulatory rise of temperature on day thirteen. Examination of her cervix showed a normal wide-open cervix on day twelve with copious clear mucus, and a closed postovulatory cervix on day fifteen. That month, her cycle was twenty-seven days, the first normal cycle she appeared to have had since discontinuing birth control pills one year earlier. The very next month, she was afraid her periods were getting irregular again, because she did not start to menstruate at twenty-eight days, but in truth she was pregnant.

The problem this couple experienced was not only an over-attention to trying to pinpoint the right day to have sex, but a disruption of her period and suppression of ovulation caused by the severe anxiety they were both under. Their experience helps explain why anywhere from 10 percent to 20 percent of infertility patients manage to get pregnant during the evaluation period, before the doctor even has a chance to institute treatment.

With other couples, the problem is that they really do not have an active enough sex life. One gynecologist has studied the frequency of sex in normal couples and related it to how long it takes for them to get pregnant. In fertile couples who have intercourse less than once a week, only 16 percent conceive within the first six months of trying. In fertile couples who have intercourse once a week, 32 percent conceive within the first six months. In fertile couples who have intercourse twice a week, 46 percent conceive within the first six months, and in those who have intercourse three times per week, 51 percent conceive within six months. Those who have intercourse four times or more a week have an 80 percent chance of pregnancy occurring within the first six months of trying. We may have to modify the recommendation of having intercourse every night, or as often as one likes, for certain patients with low sperm counts, but in general the more sex the better. Couples who have sex less than once a week are simply very unlikely to hit it at the right time, and only 16 percent are likely to get pregnant, despite the absence of any other problems, within the first six months of trying.

I have seen quite a few patients who were able to have sex only on the weekend because of heavy work schedules during the week, often involving traveling. The penalty of success in a career is sometimes a schedule so busy that intercourse, in an otherwise workable marriage, is either sporadic, or at best once a week. It takes no particular medical education to calculate that in these patients the chance of having sex at the fertile preovulatory day is one-third that of couples who have sex every other day. Furthermore, if the woman's cycle has a duration of twenty-eight days, then she is likely to be ovulating on the same particular day of the week in any given month. Thus, she may be unfortunate enough to be regularly ovulating on a Wednesday, once every four weeks, when her husband is always out of town. Of course, many couples who have sex only on the weekends have no problem impregnating, because the wife's ovulation may be occurring at that time.

Sometimes the problem with infrequent intercourse is not just a business schedule which keeps the partners apart at the appropriate time of the month, but rather a lack of interest in having intercourse more frequently. An example is a couple who had been trying unsuccessfully for several years to have children. When they told me they were having intercourse only once every two weeks, I explained to them that this was considerably less than the average, and they were a bit surprised. The husband was a very hardworking fellow who usually got home too tired to think about anything but a little quiet conversation and going to sleep. Their frequency of intercourse then did increase, and she became pregnant. Thus although a rigid schedule for intercourse is unrealistic and anxiety-provoking, at least the frequency and approximate timing of intercourse may need to be guided somewhat by an understanding of when the sexual act is more or less likely to lead to pregnancy.

Recently I saw a couple who had had no difficulty getting pregnant with their first child. However, they seemed unable to have a second child. In discussing their sexual methods, I found that while the husband was doing his military service twelve months before, the army obstetrician who took care of the wife suggested that they use a lubricant for intercourse because the wife was having a little pain with initial penetration. Most of these artificial lubricants have a detrimental effect on sperm, so I suggested that they stop using it. The very next month, she became pregnant. Cases such as this demonstrate the profound effect sexual methods can have on fertility.

## Hormone Treatment

HOSTILE CERVICAL MUCUS

A frequent cause of infertility is that the husband's sperm cannot penetrate the wife's cervical mucus. Many doctors feel that this is caused by an immunity which the wife develops to her husband's sperm. There is little solid evidence for this. You can imagine the horror that comes over a wife when she is told that she is "allergic" to her husband's sperm, and that she cannot have children because her antibodies are fighting off his sperm as though they were germs. It seems perfectly reasonable to imagine that just as viruses and bacteria stimulate our bodies to make antibodies which kill them, sperm ought to be able to evoke a similar response. In fact, the most remarkable and confusing event in all of life is that the baby, living within the mother's womb, is not re jected by the mother's antibodies, as any other foreign organism would be. The woman has some sort of poorly understood protection from mistakenly attacking her husband's sperm or the child she carries in her womb, even though in a sense these are foreign creatures, like the bacteria and the viruses which we destroy every day.

Sometimes the pronouncement that the wife is immune to her husband's sperm comes from doctors who have little training in or understanding of immunology, and is based upon laboratory tests that may be poorly controlled. In the majority of instances, "hostile" cervical mucus is not an allergic phenomenon, but is a result of either a poor hormone milieu in the woman, or poor sperm motility in the man. The mucus may only appear to be "hostile" because the man's sperm has an inadequate motility to invade it. On the other hand, the female's cervical mucus is normally "hostile" during most of the month. It is only for those few days just prior to ovulation that her cervical mucus, under the hormonal stimulation of estrogen, becomes clear enough and delicate enough to allow sperm invasion. In our experience, the majority of these cases of "hostile" mucus have not been caused by an obscure allergic reaction, but purely by lazy sperm in the male, or insufficient estrogen stimulation in the female.

A typical example is a patient I saw last summer, who had been trying for ten years to get pregnant. She finally contacted an excellent gynecologist, who evaluated her basal body temperature charts, her cervical mucus, and her husband's sperm. He found that she did not ovulate every month. The husband's sperm count was normal, but his semen contained white blood cells, suggesting an infection. Her postcoital test and cervical mucus sperm-penetration test both indicated that his sperm, despite being sufficiently motile, were not able to penetrate her cervical mucus. The doctor sent her to have sperm antibody tests performed on her blood. The antibody tests came back positive, and he sadly informed her that she had an allergy, or an immunity, to her husband's sperm.

Frequently this problem is treated by having the couple use condoms for intercourse for a period of many months, until the wife becomes less sensitive to the husband's sperm. Then when the antibody levels in her blood are lower, the couple is allowed to dismiss the condoms and hopefully the wife's immunity level will have been reduced by this period of nonexposure to his sperm. Since this patient's doctor knew that condom therapy for hostile cervical mucus was not terribly effective, he thought that first he would try at least to improve her mucus with a supplement of estrogen for four days prior to ovulation. The very first month he attempted this therapy, her cervical mucus was rapidly penetrated by her husband's sperm in large numbers, and the next month her pregnancy test was positive, after ten years of unsuccessful efforts. This case, like many others we have seen, demonstrates that looking for sperm antibodies to account for poor cervical mucus penetration is like looking for zebras in a rodeo.

The quality of cervical mucus, and the ability of sperm to penetrate it, can be improved remarkably by giving the woman 20 micrograms of estradiol (estrogen) on days ten through fourteen of her cycle. Estrogen causes the mucus to become clearer, devoid of cellular debris, softer, and thinner, so as to allow maximum sperm penetration. The rapidly rising level of estrogen on days ten through fourteen of the cycle is what normally makes the cervical mucus become penetrable during that brief period of the month. If, during that critical time, the woman's estrogen is not having sufficient effect on her cervical mucus, it makes sense to give her an estrogen supplement.

There has recently been an interest in giving women with hostile cervical mucus a course of immunosuppressive therapy (a drug called prednisone) in very high doses, with the implication that it prevents her antibodies from attacking her husband's sperm. Indeed, sperm penetration is often improved in these women, but the cause is less likely to be immunosuppressive than the fact that prednisone, like estrogen, improves the softness and clarity of the cervical mucus, making it more penetrable. Women with hostile cervical mucus often have somewhat higher levels of male hormone (testosterone) than normal. Giving prednisone to such a patient will lower her male hormone level in many instances and improve the penetrability of her cervical mucus.

I recently saw a couple who, after seven years of a barren marriage, underwent extensive immunological evaluation. They were told that she was ovulating and had normal open tubes, so the cause for her infertility had to be that her cervical mucus was hostile to her husband's sperm. Since her sperm antibody tests came back positive, they were tried on condom therapy and immunosuppressive drugs, with no improvement. When I evaluated the records, it became apparent that his sperm motility was very poor. Furthermore, her cervical mucus was not easily penetrated, even by healthy sperm, and her basal body temperature charts showed that she did not ovulate in many of her months, and ovulated late in other months. There were thus so many problems facing this particular couple (poor sperm motility of the husband, late ovulation and anovulation in the wife, insufficiently estrogenized cervical mucus, etc.) that there was no need to look for an obscure allergic phenomenon to explain their infertility. There was actually nothing I could do to help this couple, because the husband's terribly poor sperm quality could not be improved. We were able, however, by treating the wife with hormones, to improve her fertility so that she could become a candidate for artificial donor insemination.

## INDUCTION OF OVULATION

Probably the majority of women whom I see failed to conceive because they do not ovulate, or because they ovulate at irregular intervals. Although most of these women have irregular periods as a clue to their poor ovulation, it is still possible to have regular monthly periods with poor ovulation. So menstrual history, though interesting, does not really tell us enough. The greatest fertility is associated with regular, twenty-eight-day cycles, ovulation occurring precisely around day thirteen, fourteen, or fifteen. Fortunately most women with poor ovulation can be successfully treated. In the rest of this section, we will discuss the three major methods of stimulating proper ovulation.

*Prednisone.* The majority of women who do not ovulate, or who ovulate poorly, have a slightly increased amount of male hormone, testosterone, in their bloodstream. There is a great deal of unresolved medical controversy about whether this extra male hormone comes from the ovaries, from the adrenal gland, or from both. Regardless of what causes the increased production of male hormone, it is clear that this can suppress or delay ovulation, and also harm the quality of the cervical mucus. A low dose of prednisone (5 to 7 mg per day) is a very safe and effective way to reduce the woman's male hormone production in over 50 percent of these cases, and induce regular ovulation. Not only does the drop in male hormone production by the female improve the quality of ovulation, but it also improves the quality of the cervical mucus.

There is some controversy about the way in which prednisone reduces the male hormone level. The exact origin and cause of excess male hormone production in women who ovulate poorly is not really certain. There is a lot of speculation and conflicting scientific data. It appears that the excess male hormone depresses ovulation, and that lack of ovulation causes an increased production of male hormone as well.

Sometimes a combination of drugs is necessary. Prednisone may lower the male hormone level to normal, but still may not be enough to stimulate ovulation. In that case, the next drug to be discussed, Clomid, can be added to the treatment program. The two drugs together may work quite well in the difficult cases where either drug alone might not be effective.

*Clomid (Clomiphene Citrate).* For ovulation to occur, it is not sufficient merely for the pituitary gland to produce its stimulatory hormones, FSH and LH. It must produce these hormones in a specifically synchronized, properly timed fashion. The first requirement for proper ovulation is an adequate amount of FSH stimulation in the very beginning of the menstrual cycle. If there is an inadequate production of FSH by the pituitary gland right on the first day of menstruation, the early follicle may not get an adequate growth start, and this in itself sets the stage early in the cycle for poor ovulation. The object of administering the drug Clomid is to increase the pituitary's production of FSH, so that the follicle gets a good boost in the early stage of the cycle.

If the follicle gets this necessary boost by an early increase in FSH, it will develop properly and release enough estrogen around mid-cycle to trigger the pituitary gland on day fourteen to release LH, which causes the follicle to rupture and ovulate. A high level of FSH production by the pituitary gland, stimulating the follicle to grow in the early portion of the menstrual cycle, is the key to successful ovulation. The purpose of taking Clomid is to ensure that a high FSH level does occur in the early portion of the cycle. Clomid is given on days five through nine in the cycle only. It is needed just for these critical five days after the menstrual bleeding has stopped, and when maximum FSH stimulation is necessary. After day nine, Clomid is no longer needed. It has already done its job and has set the stage for the proper hormonal clockwork to take place.

Ironically, Clomid (a synthetic estrogen with very little estrogen effect) was originally introduced as a potential oral contraceptive. Researchers had hoped that this estrogen drug with no estrogen effect would suppress the pituitary's production of FSH and LH, just as modern birth control pills do. In fact, in some animals that is exactly what Clomid does. Clomid, one of the most widely used fertility drugs in the world, can actually produce infertility. Many great biological discoveries are sheer accidents, and the discovery of this remarkable drug which has brought so much happiness to women who would otherwise never have children was an accident. Rather than prevent ovulation as was originally intended, the pill has the opposite effect in humans—it stimulates ovulation.

The physician will usually start with a relatively low dose of one pill per day (50 mg) from day five to day nine of your cycle. If this does not cause you to ovulate properly, he may increase the dosage to two pills per day (100 mg), or possibly even to as high as four pills per day (200 mg). Different women respond to different doses of Clomid and that is why your doctor will usually start with a low dose. If that is effective, he will stick with it. If that dose is not effective, then he will increase it. Starting with very high doses might dangerously overstimulate the ovaries of some women. However, Clomid is generally a very safe drug and the risk of overstimulation of the ovaries is not great.

Usually, Clomid causes the follicle to develop so well that it makes enough estrogen around the mid-cycle to stimulate LH release with subsequent ovulation. However, sometimes a shot of HCG (similar to LH) is given on day fourteen to help.

To summarize, your doctor will usually give you Clomid on days five through nine, one pill per day, and if this is not sufficient, will increase the dosage to two, three, or even four pills per day. If you still do not ovulate, he may add a shot of HCG (human chorionic gonadotropin) on day fourteen or later, in an effort to get the follicle to rupture and release the egg. However, you really should respond well simply to Clomid alone.

One side effect of Clomid which can cause problems is that it frequently makes the cervical mucus too sticky to allow sperm penetration. The reason for this is that it can block the effect of estrogen on the cervix. Thus there is inadequate cervical mucus production, and even though you may be induced to ovulate properly, the sperm still cannot get in. Fortunately, the solution to this problem is fairly simple. A small dose of estrogen (simply in the form of 20 micrograms per day of ethinyl estradiol) on days ten through fourteen will usually correct any defect in the cervical mucus caused by the Clomid. Some doctors give the estrogen supplement only if they see that Clomid is hurting the cervical mucus, but other doctors give the estrogen supplement routinely, because they know that Clomid is probably exerting some influence on the cervical mucus and there is no point in allowing that side effect to get in the way of pregnancy.

Even a mild hormone like Clomid can occasionally cause excess stimulation of the ovaries, so your doctor will usually check your ovaries each month while you are menstruating before advising you to take Clomid during the next month's cycle. If on examination he finds that your ovaries are excessively enlarged, which is usually not the case with Clomid, he will advise that you omit it that month, and begin again the next month. The problem with any fertility drug, even a safe one like Clomid, is that there is not a great deal of difference between the dosage that stimulates proper ovulation and the dosage that stimulates too much ovulation.

There are two problems that occur from excess stimulation of the ovary. The first is multiple births, and the second is a complicated illness called hyperstimulation syndrome. The incidence of twins in clomiphene-treated women is about 8 percent. Triplets, quadruplets, and quintuplets are extremely rare with this relatively gentle and mild fertility agent. The complication of twins associated with this drug is frequently a welcome event.

The hyperstimulation syndrome with Clomid is usually mild, but it is potentially dangerous and should always be kept in mind. If the ovaries become significantly enlarged by hyperstimulation, then ovulation can become a rather dangerous event, leading to abdominal distention, weight gain, rapid blood-pressure drop, and severe generalized illness. This rarely occurs with Clomid, but it is seen on occasion. It can be avoided simply by omitting the drug one month, if the ovaries are too large. Your ovaries will then come down to a more normal size, so that you can undergo therapy again the following month.

At least 70 percent of women who are not ovulating at all can be induced to ovulate with Clomid and about 40 percent become pregnant within three months. The percentage of pregnancies induced for each ovulatory cycle is about 15 percent, which is not very much different from that of a normal population. The miscarriage rate is not increased above that found in a normal population of fertile women receiving no treatment. Clomid is used not only to induce ovulation in women who are not ovulating, but also to improve the quality and the regularity of ovulation. Women who ovulate on day eighteen, nineteen, or twenty without therapy will normally ovulate on day fourteen when taking Clomid. Women who have a short or inadequate luteal phase (which means that after they ovulate, their corpus luteum does not make enough progesterone and they menstruate too soon) will also become nicely regulated on Clomid. The mechanism is always the same, increased pituitary release of FSH in the early portion of the cycle, to ensure proper development of the follicle and set the stage for the precise synchrony of hormonal events to occur in the rest of the cycle.

Thus far we have discussed two very simple hormone regimens, prednisone and Clomid, which can be used by any gynecologist without the need of a sophisticated medical center. Stories of patients who have become pregnant on Clomid after years of a barren marriage are legion. In the next section, we will discuss a more drastic treatment program, which may be necessary in a small number of women who do not respond either to prednisone or Clomid.

*Pergonal.* If Clomid or prednisone fails to stimulate proper follicular growth and ovulation, a more drastic and potent hormone treatment is necessary. When Clomid fails to induce ovulation, it is usually because the pituitary gland does not respond with enough increased production of FSH. In such cases FSH must be given directly. The most commonly used brand of FSH is human menopausal gonadotropin (HMG), called Pergonal, which is made by Serono Laboratories.

Pergonal is extremely expensive. It is so potent that its dosage must be monitored almost daily by determining urinary or blood estrogen levels. These frequent tests add further to the expense. Therefore, the decision to use Pergonal in a patient whose ovulation could not be induced with prednisone or Clomid should not be taken lightly.

In the past, when Pergonal was first available, doctors did not know about the importance of monitoring daily estrogen levels, and there was a high incidence of multiple births, miscarriages, and serious hyperstimulation syndrome, with a few deaths. With modern daily monitoring of blood or urine estrogen levels, and appropriate modification of dosage, these dangerous complications have become rare. Still, 1 to 3 percent of women undergoing Pergonal therapy will get a mild degree of hyperstimulation, despite the most careful estrogen monitoring. Patients who develop this syndrome must go into the hospital, have intravenous fluids for several days, and wait for their ovaries to reduce in size and for their body to readjust.

More than 90 percent of patients can be induced to ovulate with Pergonal, and 50 percent to 70 percent will become pregnant. These are dramatic figures, since the group of patients who receive Pergonal could not possibly have conceived without it. Anywhere from 10 percent to 25 percent of the pregnancies are multiple births which are usually twins, but can sometimes be triplets, quadruplets, quintuplets, or even sextuplets. These women require a great deal of FSH activity to stimulate the follicles to develop, and when they do develop, the excess stimulation frequently results in more than one ripe ovulation during the month.

Pergonal will only prepare the follicles to be ripe for ovulation, which must be induced at the appropriate time by a separate injection of HCG. If the ovaries develop too rapidly and the estrogen level climbs out of control, it is a warning that it would be dangerous for this woman to ovulate. As long as she is not given her HCG injection at mid-cycle, the woman will not develop hyperstimulation syndrome. She can then be given a month or so to rest, and her ovaries will shrink back to a more normal size. But if she is given HCG when her ovaries are too enlarged, the follicles may have reached enormous proportions, producing inordinate amounts of estrogen, and the ovulation induced by HCG would be an intra-abdominal catastrophe that could even kill her. Despite severe ovarian enlargement, she will be in no danger as long as HCG is not administered.

The inherent dangers of Pergonal can be controlled by monitoring the woman's estrogen levels and withholding the HCG injection if her estrogen should climb too rapidly to too high a level. Some laboratories will monitor the estrogen level in the urine, and others will do a rapid test for estrogen in the blood. The blood estrogen level is a little more convenient because the answer is obtained much more quickly (usually within four hours). Normally the woman would have her blood tested for estrogen each day as she approaches the mid-cycle. The Pergonal would not be given on any day until the report came back showing that her estrogen was not already too high. When her estrogen was at the right level, she would be ready to receive HCG to induce ovulation.

The history of patients who required Pergonal to become pregnant is always exciting, because these patients would have had no hope otherwise. Their ovaries were terribly resistant to ovulation and only the maximal FSH stimulation could get them pregnant. Women who successfully become pregnant on Pergonal usually have no regrets, despite the extraordinary cost and risk.

The Serono drug company, which makes Pergonal, has collected a series of typical cases demonstrating the proper use of the drug. One classic example is a thirty-year-old woman who had been on oral contraceptives from ages twenty-two to twenty-six and did not resume ovulation after the pills were discontinued. Treatment with estrogen and progesterone accomplished nothing, and evaluation of her tubes showed no obstruction. Her husband's semen analysis was completely normal. Even the maximum doses of Clomid (up to 250 mg per day) in addition to ten thousand units of HCG could not induce her to ovulate. As soon as Pergonal was instituted, she began to ovulate and after five cycles of treatment she finally became pregnant. She gave birth nine months later to a normal boy.

Another patient was a twenty-nine-year-old woman who was married at the age of twenty-three, but at age twenty-six had to undergo surgery for blocked tubes, which was felt to be a cause of her infertility. She became pregnant shortly thereafter, and now three years later was once again trying to have another baby. Her basal body temperatures did demonstrate ovulation, but the ovulation occurred late, irregularly, and was associated with a short luteal phase. The patient was treated with Clomid for six months, up to 150 mg per day for five days, and her temperature charts improved moderately, but she still did not become pregnant. Even after three months of Clomid plus HCG, she failed to achieve pregnancy.

As a last resort, she was placed on Pergonal in the same fashion as women who are not ovulating at all. Her scanty cervical mucus suddenly became more copious and after nine days of treatment, when her urinary estrogens reached good levels, an ovulatory dose of HCG was given. After this one cycle of Pergonal and HCG she became pregnant and delivered a normal child. This particular case demonstrates that there are some difficult patients who appear to ovulate but have defects in their cycle with poor-quality ovulation and even Clomid may not be effective in treating them. These unusual cases also can be helped by Pergonal.

In another case, a twenty-seven-year-old woman with four years of infertility had undergone surgery of the left ovary for endometriosis and later a complete removal of the left ovary and tube. The patient then underwent further surgery to release scar tissue which was holding down the only remaining tube and preventing it from grasping any egg that might have ovulated. After the operation, the patient showed poor maturation of the follicle, inadequate cervical mucus, and a short luteal phase. Treatment with estrogen, HCG, and extra progesterone in the luteal phase did not improve ovulation. Clomid caused a marked improvement in the temperature chart, but the cervical mucus remained scanty and thick. Estrogens were therefore used in addition to Clomid in order to improve the cervical mucus. She still did not get pregnant until she was given Pergonal for nine days followed by ten thousand units of HCG. After three months of this treatment, she finally conceived and had a normal pregnancy.

Thus, although Pergonal should be considered a last resort in patients with poor ovulation or no ovulation, it may sometimes be necessary in situations where one might have expected Clomid or prednisone to be sufficient therapy. The failure of Clomid to regulate what might be thought of as only a mild ovulatory defect is sufficient indication to use Pergonal.

*Bromocryptine.* Occasionally a lack of ovulation is caused by increased levels of a hormone called prolactin, which is released by the pituitary normally after the delivery of a baby to allow breast-feeding. Prolactin directly stimulates the breasts to make milk. It also prevents ovulation. In some patients a small and otherwise undetectable pituitary tumor may cause the prolactin level in the blood to be increased, and make them infertile. Although this is a new and controversial subject, a drug called Bromocryptine, which is available in Canada and Europe but has not yet been formally released for use in the United States, dramatically suppresses the pituitary's production of prolactin in these cases and ovulation ensues promptly after its administration. Bromocryptine is not useful in other cases of infertility and is not a cure-all fertility drug. However, it is an exciting new treatment for women who are found on routine screening for infertility to have increased production of prolactin.

What to do about the pituitary tumor itself and whether or not it requires surgical treatment are outside the scope of this book. With newer microsurgical techniques neurosurgeons are making this sort of pituitary surgery much safer than it has been in the past, and more and more women may be undergoing this operation in the future. Nonetheless, controversy exists as to whether or not the tumor should be left alone. Certainly Bromocryptine will eventually have to be accepted by the FDA for usage in the United States, and then at least there will be a choice.

*Ovarian Wedge Resection.* One rather crude form of therapy used in the past for women who do not ovulate is the surgical removal of a portion of their ovaries. This barbaric-sounding approach actually had a significant success rate. Although not recommended today because of the excellent drugs available to induce ovulation, such surgery was moderately successful in the past, and tells us a little bit about why these ovaries do not ovulate. The only important and documented hormonal change in non-ovulating women who have undergone ovarian wedge resection is that their blood testosterone levels drop dramatically. This suggests that the high production of testosterone by the ovary is one of the reasons why follicles are not forming properly and not ovulating. A wedge resection is a bit like hitting an ovary over the head and temporarily preventing it from making hormones. When the male hormone production of the ovary is thus stopped, ovulatory cycles frequently resume. The problems with this surgery are that it causes potentially harmful scar tissue around the ovary, and that it does not solve the problem permanently. Most patients again fail to ovulate after a certain period of time has passed. Thus ovarian wedge resection is now becoming a treatment of the past.

## Scarred Tubes

Another major component of the woman's fertility is the ability of her fallopian tubes to grasp the egg from the ovary at the time of ovulation, draw it in, provide a healthy environment for fertilization to occur, and then, after several days of development, transport the embryo into the womb to be implanted. For this complicated series of events to take place, the tube must be unobstructed and freely mobile. Any scars on the inside which block the passageway, or scars on the outside which limit the tube's range of movement, can prevent proper transport of the egg, and result in the severest and most difficult sort of infertility to treat. The most common cause of such tubal scarring is infection. Often the infection may have gone completely undetected, and finally burned itself out in the form of a scar. At least half of the women we see with this problem have no real recollection of any symptoms to suggest infection, although we know this has to be the origin of the scar in most instances.

The two tests which allow the gynecologist to determine whether this problem exists are the hysterosalpingogram (an X ray of the tubes) and laparoscopy. The X ray indicates what area of the tube is blocked. External scarring of the tube, which hinders its mobility, is best determined by laparoscopy— actually viewing the tubes and the ovary through a telescope. Laparoscopy requires a brief hospitalization, and therefore is generally not performed until the doctor is sure that all other aspects of fertility have been evaluated. These two tests are both somewhat uncomfortable. Neither one of the tests alone is sufficient to tell the gynecologist what he or she needs to know about the functioning of the tubes. Both tests are usually necessary before any surgical treatment can be contemplated, either to release the scarring or to open up the obstruction.

The most favorable type of scarring to treat surgically is the kind that blocks the mobility of the tube on the outside, rather than the kind that has destroyed portions of the internal lining. You will recall that the lining of the tube has little cilia that beat at a rate of twelve hundred times per minute toward the uterus, to help draw the egg into the tube. Without the delicate function of these billions of cilia lining the tube, the egg could not be transported. Even though modern surgical techniques will allow an internally obstructed tube to be reopened, poor functioning of the cilia may still prevent pregnancy. On the other hand, if the scarring is limited to the outside of the tube, the cilia usually are not badly damaged, and simply freeing the tube from the scar tissue that has held it in place will result in over a 50-percent pregnancy rate.

When the scarring is located inside the tube, it is usually densest at the very end, with the fimbria completely closed off.

Thus none of the tube communicates any longer with the abdominal cavity. The fluid secreted into the tube builds up pressure, and such a tube is blown up almost like a balloon. As a result of this, the lining of the tube undergoes a great deal of damage, and surgical reopening of the fimbria (an operation called salpingostomy), still results in only a 30-percent pregnancy rate in the very best surgical hands.

When an infection that occurred many years ago causes scarring and blockage to occur at the canal that joins the tube to the uterus, rather than at the fimbrial end of the tube, there is no such buildup of pressure and the cilia are not damaged. Modern microsurgical techniques can open up this obstruction quite elegantly, and pregnancy rates of up to 80 percent can be achieved. Unfortunately, most of the cases of scarring and blockage of the tubes that we see occur at the fimbriated end, and no matter how elegant the surgery, the pregnancy rate is not likely to exceed 30 percent in such patients.

### Endometriosis

Endometriosis is a very common disorder, found in up to 20 percent of infertile women, in which the endometrial tissue which normally lines the uterus grows in other areas of the abdominal cavity, usually surrounding the ovaries and the tubes. Though endometriosis is in many respects a mysterious condition, most authorities believe it is caused by a portion of the menstrual flow traveling backward through the tubes into the body cavity rather than forward out through the cervix and vagina. When the menstrual flow regurgitates backward into the abdominal cavity, some of the endometrial tissue can gain a foothold there and begin to grow and develop just as though it were in the womb. Endometriosis can be massive or tiny. It can attach to the tubes, the ovaries, or to the lining of the abdominal wall.

These implants bleed whenever menstruation occurs, just as they would if they were in the uterus. During menstruation, blood comes out of the cervix and vagina because of the shedding of the uterine lining. With endometriosis the same process takes place inside the abdomen, but in these locations the blood cannot drain out of the body. Thus with every menstrual period there is an inordinate amount of pain, and gradually over the years scarring and distortion of the normal architecture of the tubes and ovaries occur.

Endometriosis is a very common disorder, which seems to be occurring with greater frequency in the modern era. In societies where girls marry young and have babies early in life, the condition is much less common. It seems that the more menstrual periods a woman has, the greater is her chance of eventually developing endometriosis. During each menstrual cycle, there is a chance of a few cells of the uterine lining going backward, up the fallopian tubes. Girls begin to menstruate now much earlier in life than they did two hundred years ago, probably because of better nutrition. Then they put off childbearing for many years. Thus, the modern woman experiences many more menstrual periods than did her predecessors.

The two major symptoms of endometriosis are inordinately painful periods and infertility. Many women who are infertile because of endometriosis have relatively little pain during their periods and many women with painful periods have no endometriosis, and no difficulty getting pregnant. Although a gynecologist's suspicion is always aroused by the complaint of infertility and very painful menstrual periods, endometriosis can exist with either one or with neither of these symptoms.

The only way to establish a firm diagnosis of endometriosis is to perform a laparoscopy. Frequently endometrial implants are detected by this procedure even though they were not suspected originally to be the cause of infertility.

NATURE'S CURES FOR ENDOMETRIOSIS

It is ironic that pregnancy, which endometriosis helps to prevent, is also the best cure for the disease. The enormous and steady increase in progesterone during the nine months of pregnancy usually destroys most of the endometrial implants more successfully than any other treatment available. The problem is that the distortion of genital architecture caused by endometriosis interferes with the chances of getting pregnant. Once pregnancy is achieved, however, the constant stimulation of progesterone, though initially causing the implants to swell somewhat, eventually results in their drying up. It is the cyclic, monthly growth and shedding of the endometrial tissue which stimulates its enlargement and causes most of the problems.

Another natural cure for endometriosis is menopause. When the ovaries finally shed their last egg and the production of estrogen and progesterone diminishes, the lining of the uterus begins to dry up, and so do the endometrial implants. The severest forms of endometriosis will be cured eventually by menopause. That is a long time to wait, however, and if you have not been able to have children in the interim, the condition will have taken its tragic toll. Fortunately, by understanding that pregnancy and menopause are both cures for the disorder, doctors have been able to develop hormonal treatments that mimic these conditions temporarily, and thus destroy the endometriosis almost as effectively. When hormonal treatment does not seem sufficient because of permanent scarring that persists after the endometriosis is destroyed, surgery to release these scarred areas can help even further.

There are two effective hormonal methods of treating endometriosis, one of which mimics pregnancy and the other menopause. Both methods are designed to prevent monthly menstruation, thus allowing the endometrial implants to disintegrate. The effect of both treatments on the uterine lining is the same. The hope is that after about three to nine months of such hormonal treatment, the endometrial implants will have dried up permanently. However, the lining of the uterus, the natural place where endometrium should grow, will always redevelop after treatment is discontinued.

## ARTIFICIAL PREGNANCY

The most time-honored treatment for endometriosis is to induce the hormonal equivalent of pregnancy. Birth control pills are taken every day for as long as nine months. Unlike when birth control pills are used to prevent pregnancy, however (when the pills are taken for three weeks of the cycle), in this case the pills are taken every day. This presents the body with a continuous rather than a periodic burst of estrogen and progesterone to prevent menstruation, much like what occurs in pregnancy. During the first two or three months of treatment, there may be more pain. However, after that time there will be a gradual drying up of the endometrial implants, just as though pregnancy had occurred before such treatment was required. Up to 90 percent of patients have marked improvement in symptoms from this treatment, and more than 50 percent will be able to become pregnant after the therapy is discontinued. It may seem odd that oral contraceptives can actually improve fertility, but of course one cannot get pregnant until the treatment is discontinued and ovulation begins.

## ARTIFICIAL MENOPAUSE

The second method of hormonal treatment for endometriosis, which is much more recently available, is to produce a false menopause. Until recently, the complete and temporary suppression of the ovaries' production of hormones could not be achieved medically. Any hormones capable of stopping the pituitary gland from secreting FSH and LH also had strong male or female hormonal side effects. Now, however, there is a relatively expensive new pill called Danazol, which completely blocks FSH and LH production by the pituitary and thus temporarily produces a false menopause. Four tablets are taken daily for an average of six months. Shortly after this medication is begun, ovulation and menstruation will stop. Mild menopausal symptoms such as hot flashes and night sweats may even develop. Only a few patients have these side effects, however, and they are usually mild.

After treatment with Danazol is discontinued, regular menstrual periods begin to return within four to six weeks. Almost all patients have relief of symptoms with this treatment. Seventy-two percent of patients who were otherwise infertile are able to conceive following this treatment. About 30 percent of patients eventually have a recurrence of symptoms. If the disorder recurs, it usually does so in the second half of the first year after the drug is discontinued. If endometriosis has not recurred after the first year of stopping the drug, there is only a 5 percent chance of its recurring with each succeeding year. On the bright side, over 60 percent of patients who take Danazol are permanently cured and require no reinstitution of therapy. The improvement in symptoms and the restoration of fertility with this drug are quite remarkable.

Since Danazol induces a "false" menopause and prevents the ovaries from releasing the female hormones estrogen and progesterone, you might naturally ask what effect this treatment will have on your sex life during the six months that you must be subjected to it. Actually the sex drive is slightly increased with Danazol because it has a very weak male hormone activity. You will remember that humans, unlike most other animals, derive their sex drive in both males and females from the male hormone, testosterone. Castration of the human female (that is, removal of ovaries) does not cause reduction in sex drive, even though in most lower animals it prevents the periodic occurrence of heat and puts a permanent and drastic end to sexual activity. Danazol seems to produce for women the ideal situation of not having to worry about menstruation and yet suffering no reduction in sexual interest.

Very large endometrial lesions may have to be removed surgically, on occasion. In addition, scarring left after the endometriosis has disappeared may require surgery as well. Usually when the endometriosis is controlled by hormone treatment, there is sufficient restoration of a normal genital environment for pregnancy to occur. However, the scarring that surrounds the endometrial implants can sometimes be of such magnitude that the tubes and the uterus remain distorted, and in this case surgery will be needed to release their entrapment.

There is a great deal of controversy among gynecologists as to whether surgery or hormonal treatment is the best approach to curing endometriosis. There is no disagreement that scarring left in the wake of endometriosis may need to be treated surgically. The big question is whether large endometrial implants need to be removed with the surgeon's knife or are best treated with hormonal suppression. One problem with being too aggressive surgically is that the very surgery designed to remove the endometrial implants may sometimes create more adhesion, scarring, and entrapment of the ovaries and tubes than did the original endometriosis. There is no clear-cut answer to this dilemma, and each woman must be treated individually. But at least now there are powerful hormonal tools for dealing with this very mysterious and aggravating cause of infertility.

## Microsurgery and Reversal of Tubal Sterilization

Tubal sterilization is now even more popular than vasectomy in this country as a method of permanent birth control. It is estimated that over a half million women undergo tubal ligation each year. One reason for the dramatic increase in popularity of this procedure is the use of the laparoscope, which makes it possible to sterilize a woman through a tiny incision less than one-half inch long in the belly-button area. A woman need not spend more than a day in the hospital, and she has minimal discomfort. Despite the fact that women are warned that sterilization is a permanent procedure, a certain small percentage change their minds and decide they would like to have more children. With previous surgical techniques, only 5 percent to 20 percent of these women could possibly have had their fertility restored. With modern microsurgery, however, this tiny tube can be accurately put together again in almost every instance, and up to 80 percent of these women can then have more children. This delicate microsurgery is performed properly only by a small number of doctors at the present time. It requires a great deal of practice and patience, using high-power magnification and thread that is essentially invisible to the naked eye to put together properly a tube whose inner diameter in some areas can be as tiny as a pinpoint (see Fig. 16).

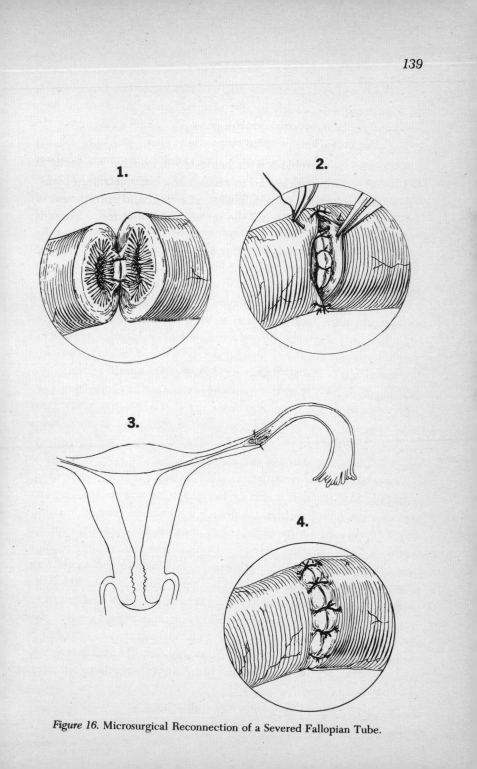

*Figure 16.* Microsurgical Reconnection of a Severed Fallopian Tube.

Thanks to new microsurgical techniques, we are now able to help men and women whose decision to be sterilized would have been tragically irreversible in the past. A typical case involved a twenty-three-year-old woman who had been sterilized at age twenty. She had already had two pregnancies terminated by abortion and was in a state of panic, when a physician agreed to tie her tubes. Three years later her whole life changed: she was happily married, in a very stable situation, and regretted her impetuous decision at age twenty to prevent herself from ever getting pregnant again. The first gynecologist she saw told her there was too little tube to work with, but sent her to us to see whether a microsurgical approach might be possible. When we explored her abdomen, indeed we did find that a very large amount of tube had been destroyed by the sterilization procedure, but there still was some tube left to work with. We were able to reconnect it very accurately to the tiny opening which leads into the womb. X rays taken six weeks later showed that the tubes were properly reconnected, and our major worry at that point was whether her tubes would be long enough to grasp the egg from the surface of the ovary. One year later her pregnancy test was positive. She went on to deliver a normal little baby.

Not all such women are so fortunate. We have seen many women (about 5 percent) whose sterilization procedure was so destructive that the fimbriated end of the tube was destroyed. Last year I received a letter from a doctor who was writing on behalf of his sister in her mid-twenties, who wanted very much to have a child. While in her late teens she became pregnant out of wedlock, and allegedly was told that she would only be allowed an abortion if she also agreed to have a tubal ligation. Six years later she had a happy, stable marriage, loved to play with children and take care of them, was able to pay any kind of hospital or surgical fee, and would have been willing to undergo any treatment in order to be able to get pregnant. Unfortunately her fimbria had been completely removed, along with most of her tubes, and there was nothing we could do for her.

A very stable thirty-two-year-old woman married to a thirty-five-year-old man for several years came to see us. Her husband had two children from a previous marriage, and he had been vasectomized during that marriage. She had three children from a previous marriage, and had had her tubes tied during that marriage. Neither one of them would have predicted that their marriages would fall apart several years after their respective sterilizations. Now that they were both happily remarried, they wished to have more children but they didn't dream this could possibly be achieved. However, with the dramatic improvement in results that we have been able to achieve with microsurgery, we knew the chances would be excellent. We first reversed her tubal ligation, and then reversed his vasectomy. There was only about an inch and a half of her tube left on each side, so we were somewhat concerned about the short length of her remaining tube. The operative results were beautiful, but we did not know whether the tube would be long enough to catch the egg. A year later we reversed her husband's vasectomy. He recovered a normal sperm count after three months; shortly thereafter, she became pregnant, and nine months later she delivered a healthy little baby.

With the older methods of reversing tubal ligations, there was a high risk of ectopic pregnancy. This was because the passageway which was restored between the two disconnected ends of the tube was not a normal passageway, and the egg would frequently get caught on its way into the uterus. It would then develop and grow in the tube instead of the womb. It would rupture in the tube and die, requiring surgical removal. This risk, although present, is minimal with modern microsurgical techniques, which establish a more reliable passageway between the severed ends of the tube. If the amount of tube destroyed by sterilization procedure is small, almost all who desire it are able to have their fertility restored with microsurgery.

The major stumbling block for these patients is that a significant number of them have had an unnecessarily large amount of tube destroyed, in an effort to make the sterilization definitive. If instead only a tiny segment, perhaps a half inch of the tube, were burned or destroyed in the process of severing it, almost all women so sterilized would be able to achieve pregnancy again after undergoing a microsurgical reconnection. Although women in their middle or late thirties may do best with a more destructive sterilization procedure that has a poor chance for reversal, young girls who seem to be caught in the dilemma of too many pregnancies too early in life, or women who are experiencing marital difficulties, or are single, might prefer to have a minimally destructive sterilization procedure so as to keep their future options a bit more open.

# ·5·

# Treatment of the Male

When a couple was unable to have children, physicians used to decide all too quickly that it was either the husband's or the wife's fault. If the husband's sperm count was low, the couple was told that it was his fault, and treatment would be directed only toward him. If his sperm count was high, they were told it was the wife's fault. We now know that infertility is usually a combination of problems in the husband and in the wife. A man with a low sperm count can frequently impregnate a very fertile woman, even though he could not impregnate a relatively infertile woman. On the other hand, a man with a very high sperm count can often impregnate a woman who is not very fertile. We can't really say what is a normal sperm count, but to increase the statistical likelihood of pregnancy the higher the sperm count the better.

In some cases of male infertility there has been spectacular progress, as with the man who has been vasectomized, or the man with a varicose vein of the testicle. However, in many cases, efforts to improve the man's sperm count fail, and in such cases the best treatment is to maximize the wife's fertility. There is such a bewildering array of unproven, witchcraftlike remedies to which infertile men may be subjected that every infertile male should read this chapter before accepting such treatment.

## Varicose Veins of the Testicle

HOW DOES A VARICOSE VEIN CAUSE INFERTILITY?

About 10 percent of all men have a large, swollen varicose vein (varicocele) on the left testicle. A varicose vein of the testicle is just like a varicose vein of the leg. When you stand up, the veins fill with blood draining down from the rest of the body. Blood can normally only make its way back to the heart because of valves all along the way that prevent backflow. Much like the steps of a ladder, they allow returning blood to make its way slowly toward the heart even while we are standing up. When these retaining valves are damaged, blood falls back downward toward the lower half of the body, especially when we stand. It cannot easily make its way back unless we lie down again. In fact, the only way that blood can get back while we are standing is by detouring through other, collateral veins that do have properly functioning valves.

Varicose veins of the legs are unsightly and irritating, but blood usually finds its way back through deeper veins. Sometimes, however, so much blood is regurgitated back down toward the legs that swelling and aching discomfort can occur. It is common for such patients to require corrective surgery. A varicose vein of the testicle works in much the same way. It is so frequently found in normal men that for many years it was not even considered an abnormality. We now know that it is one of the most common treatable causes of male infertility. In most men, a varicocele does not seem to cause infertility. However, in men who are infertile and who have a varicocele, surgery has a 70 percent to 80 percent chance of significantly improving the sperm count, and over a 50 percent chance of resulting in pregnancy.

Why should some men with a varicocele be fertile and others not? Why does varicocele occur almost always on the left side? How does varicocele hurt sperm production? Why aren't all men who have a varicocele infertile? If varicocele usually occurs only on the left side, why should both testicles be affected? Varicocele is still a big puzzle to scientists and doctors in the field of fertility.

First, you should know why the varicocele is most commonly on the left side rather than the right. The major vein that drains blood from the left testicle travels a very long distance, all the way up to the kidneys, inside the abdomen, and only at that relatively high level empties into a major trunk. The veins of almost every other part of the body have a much shorter distance to travel. Oddly enough, the left testicular vein travels a much longer distance than the right testicular vein. This difference in anatomy between the left and the right sides causes the valves on the left to break down more frequently, and a varicose vein of the left testicle to occur. Varicose veins of the testicle do not develop gradually with age, as do varicose veins of the leg. Rather, they appear during puberty, when testicular blood flow increases. People do not generally develop them later in life.

Why should a varicose vein on the left side affect sperm production on both sides? Actually, it usually affects sperm production in the left testicle more than the right. In addition, the stagnation of blood which the varicose vein causes on the left can easily cross over to the right, and therefore affect both sides. That is why operating only on the side that has the varicose vein can improve the sperm production on both sides. Since we know that 20 percent to 40 percent of infertile men have a varicose vein of their testicle, and 10 percent of fertile men have one also, we have to ask why varicocele seems to be harmful to some men and not to others. Scientists don't know the answer for sure, but there are a number of theories. Which particular theory we accept can influence whether literally millions of men during the next ten years are asked to undergo surgery for a varicocele that may be doing them no harm whatsoever.

There are three basic theories: (1) the testicles are too warm from all this backward-flowing blood; (2) stagnation of blood in the varicose vein creates poor circulation of oxygen and nutrients to the testicle; and (3) hormones produced higher up in the abdomen by the adrenal gland pass downward into the testicle and inhibit sperm production. The heat theory is the most popular. In just about all animals except for the elephant, the rhinoceros, and the whale, normal body temperature prevents sperm production and can damage the testicle. The reason that the testicles are located outside of the body in the scrotal sac is that the temperature there is four degrees lower than the body temperature. Men who are born with testicles in their abdomen, which are not later surgically brought into the scrotum, will not produce sperm. Similarly, if warm abdominal blood is constantly draining backward into the scrotum through a testicular varicose vein, the temperature in the scrotum might be elevated sufficiently to impede sperm production. There is a complicated heat-exchange mechanism designed to keep the testicular temperature always about four degrees Fahrenheit below the rest of the body. This involves a very long, but tiny, testicular artery carrying warm blood from the abdomen, running alongside the vein that is returning cooler blood back from the testicle. This warm arterial blood is cooled off by the blood returning via the testicular veins. A varicose vein with stagnant blood would interfere with this temperature-regulating mechanism in the scrotum, and allow too high a temperature for proper sperm production.

A number of scientists have actually measured the scrotal temperature in infertile subjects with varicocele and compared it with the scrotal temperature of normal men. The scrotal temperature of infertile men with varicocele has been found to be about one and one-half degrees Fahrenheit warmer than the scrotal temperature of normal men. Doctors in Belgium have used a technique called thermography to actually photograph the temperature elevation in the testicles of infertile men with varicocele. This technique involves taking a picture of the scrotum with an infrared camera which picks up differences in temperature rather than light on photographic film. By looking at such an infrared picture, they can determine which men have warm testicles and which men have cool testicles. Almost all of the men with varicose veins had warm testicles. All of the normal men without varicocele had cool testicles.

Many of the infertile men in whom no varicose veins could be detected on physical examination were also found to have warm testicles, suggesting to the Belgian scientists that the infertility of these men may be due to a varicose vein undetectable on physical examination but which is still doing its subtle damage to the man's fertility. If these studies are verified, it could mean that not only will all men with varicocele be operated on regardless of whether they are presently infertile, but also all men who are infertile will be operated on regardless of whether they have a varicocele. In fact, this very approach is now being used in Denmark, and has been seriously recommended by some doctors in the United States for all infertile men. This potential epidemic of scrotal surgery (which may have some economic force behind it) may well cause all concerned men to shudder.

Another theory about varicocele is that hormones may pass down from the kidney area through the testicular vein, and thus inhibit sperm production directly. Most scientists who have measured hormone concentrations in the testicular blood of varicocele patients and normal patients have not found any firm evidence to support this theory.

The third way in which a varicose vein is thought to harm the testicle is that the stagnation of blood returning through the vein from the testicle could interfere with proper circulation of blood nutrients and oxygen. Certainly men and women with varicose veins of the leg often develop aching, swelling, and even skin damage, because of the stagnation of blood. It has nothing to do with temperature regulation or hormones, but simply interference with proper circulation caused by inability of the blood to get back properly while the person is standing. Sluggish blood flow to the testicles caused by the stagnant varicose vein could result in decreased delivery of oxygen and nutrients.

Regardless of how varicocele contributes to male infertility, the puzzle still remains: why are most men with varicocele fertile? If a varicocele is left untreated in a young man, might his future fertility be jeopardized? Varicocele may be harmful to every man's fertility, but some are just luckier than others. Patients whose varicoceles are causing infertility may be those who started out with a low sperm count which worsened because of the varicocele. Fertile men in their twenties who wish to put off having children for another ten years may find themselves sterile later because of a varicocele that had been considered harmless.

## THE OPERATION AND ITS EFFECT ON SPERM COUNT

What sort of operation does an infertile man with varicose vein of the testicle have to undergo? Actually it is not a very big operation, and in good hands not one to be terribly worried about. All of the little testicular veins draining the testicle converge into one or two veins a little higher up in the lower part of the abdomen. A relatively small incision is made in this area. It looks just like an appendectomy incision except that it is on the left side instead of the right side, and does not go beneath the abdominal wall. The vein or veins in this region are occluded by tying them with a simple piece of surgical thread and then dividing them. After the operation, blood from the abdomen can no longer flow down under the influence of gravity, and blood leaving the testicle returns to the body through collateral routes. This operation requires no more than one or two days in the hospital, and involves minimal discomfort. Afterward, when the patient stands, the left of his scrotum will no longer fill up with blood.

Seventy to 80 percent of patients have a significant improvement in their sperm count afterward, but this is not noticed until three months or more after the operation. The reason for this delay is that it takes sperm about three months to be manufactured and then released in the ejaculate. Thus any improvement in sperm production caused by the operation will only be noticeable after three months have passed. Most doctors report that 40 to 60 percent of the infertile men whom they treat for varicocele will eventually impregnate their wives after the operation.

Not all infertile men have the same outlook for success after the varicocele operation. In patients whose sperm counts are initially under ten million per cc, only 30 percent will impregnate their wives, and their improvement in sperm count is less likely to be significant. In patients whose sperm count is initially over ten million per cc, up to 60 percent will impregnate their wives, and their improvement in sperm count after the operation is much more likely to be dramatic. Patients with varicocele who have no sperm in their ejaculate before the operation have a very low chance of success, but occasionally spectacular results can be achieved even in these cases. In fact, the very first documented report of success with this operation for varicocele was of a man who started out with no sperm at all. The operation took place in England in April 1950. The patient was a twenty-seven year old who had absolutely no sperm in his ejaculate, and his testicle biopsy showed severe failure of sperm production. He had very large varicose veins not only on the left testicle but also on the right. Six months after surgery his sperm count had risen from zero up to eighteen million per cc, and by one year the sperm count was twenty-seven million per cc. His wife soon became pregnant and delivered a normal child.

This first successful case of restoration of fertility after varicocelectomy stimulated widespread interest in what appears to be one of the most effective treatments for male infertility. But ironically the chances for that particular first patient's having a successful operation were very slim, because he started out in the worst possible category (complete absence of sperm). For the next ten years surgeons in America remained skeptical and dubious about the role of this operation in helping infertile men, even though encouraging reports continued to come across the Atlantic from outstanding fertility experts in Britain. It wasn't until the early 1960s that American fertility experts began to endorse this operation for their patients.

## THE WIFE'S ROLE WHEN HER HUSBAND HAS VARICOCELE

Despite our enthusiasm for correcting varicocele in infertile men, the major problem is sometimes not the varicocele, or indeed the husband's marginal sperm count, but a problem in the wife that goes undetected simply because the husband has a varicocele. It has been demonstrated conclusively that if, instead of performing surgery on the husband, doctors treat the wife to maximize *her* fertility, the pregnancy rate is equivalent to that achieved by treating the man's varicocele. Certainly surgery to correct varicocele does raise the sperm count, and in some men raises it sufficiently to increase greatly their chances of impregnating their spouses. On the other hand, in the majority of cases a significant fertility problem in the wife is neglected because of overattention to the husband's varicocele.

A young man was referred to me several years ago because of a low sperm count: only twenty-five million per cc with motility of only 25 percent. He had been trying unsuccessfully to impregnate his wife for the last two years. Without any physical examination, a urologist had placed him on thyroid medication, an approach which has fallen completely into disrepute. Of course this had no effect on his sperm count and he was finally referred to me. When I detected an obvious varicocele on physical examination, I simply assumed that the reason for the continued barrenness of their marriage was the neglect of the previous urologist in not finding this varicocele and operating on it. After I operated on the patient, his sperm count increased to eighty million per cc and the motility went up to 90 percent. We had dramatically improved his sperm count with a single operation, and I felt it would just be a matter of time before he and his wife had that child they wanted so badly.

All along, the wife had been assured by her gynecologist that she was fertile, but I didn't realize that the husband's low sperm count had dulled her gynecologist's enthusiasm for evaluating her carefully. It wasn't until a year later when she was still not pregnant that I insisted that she be reevaluated. We then discovered that in truth she was not ovulating properly, and after therapy with Clomid she conceived and had a normal pregnancy. I had been so enthusiastic when we discovered the cause of the husband's infertility that I neglected to check the wife to make sure we were not missing something obvious in her. Of course the dramatic improvement in his sperm count increased their chances for pregnancy, and the operation was probably not a waste, but I had completely neglected the most important factor in their barren marriage.

Another patient of mine had been trying for eleven years to impregnate his wife, with no success. They already had one adopted child whom they were able to obtain before adoption became so difficult. The husband's sperm count was fifty million per cc with 50 percent motility, but because of a varicocele he was referred to me for infertility. The wife did not want to come to the appointment because she had already been assured by her gynecologist ten years before that she was fine, and also because she was having her period that day and was very uncomfortable. Indeed, she was having severe menstrual cramps and gave a history dating back many years of very painful, heavy periods typical of endometriosis. Examination did in fact reveal endometriosis, which was the true cause of their infertility, rather than the husband's varicocele. The surgeon can easily rush in with his knife to cure a varicocele, but the varicocele may not really be the main culprit.

## RISKS OF OPERATING ON THE VARICOCELE

Not only can other causes of infertility be mistakenly neglected in a patient with a varicocele, but the operation itself on occasion may produce more harm than good. I have already seen several patients who prior to having a varicocelectomy elsewhere had excellent sperm counts, but who after the operation were sterile. These were unusual cases in which the varicocele was on both the left and the right sides. The artery supplying the testicle runs very close to the varicose vein, and it was inadvertently tied off with the vein. If this were to happen in the usual varicocele operation, no obvious untoward result would be observed, because the unoperated testicle would remain unscathed. However, when the operation is necessary on both sides, there is a definite risk of causing more harm than good.

This operation is considered easy by most surgeons. They often don't realize how very tiny is the artery supplying the testicle (about one-seventh of an inch in diameter). It is terribly easy for it to be damaged unless very delicate techniques are used to safeguard it. We usually get along with crude techniques in this very common operation because it is performed most often on one side only, and because there is often a good collateral arterial blood supply coming to the testicles from other arteries that are not damaged. But sometimes the collateral circulation is not very good. I have even seen one young man who became a eunuch after this "harmless" operation.

Another disaster I have recently seen following a varicocele operation can serve as a grim reminder of what problems may lie ahead if doctors do indeed decide that all young men with varicocele require an early operation. I received a consultation from a very nice urologist in another community who had apparently gotten into hot water. He had performed a varicocelectomy on a teenager with no known fertility problem. The varicocele was so large that he felt it would be wise to operate on it at this very early stage. He sadly confessed that a segment of the vas deferens was inadvertently removed. The doctor's intentions in performing the operation were good, but the result was frightening.

These notes of caution about varicocelectomy are only intended to give an in-depth understanding of a problem which may face up to 20 percent of young men in the world. I do not mean to diminish the importance of treating a varicocele in infertile couples. Varicocelectomy remains one of the most effective methods of curing male infertility, and is likely to be performed in 30 percent of couples who are having difficulty with conception. I only caution that we should not jump into a varicocele operation so blindly that we neglect other problems that may be equally important causes of the couple's infertility.

## Vasectomy Reversal and Microsurgery

Vasectomy is one of the most common operations performed today in the United States, and it is the most popular method of birth control in the world. At least ten million American men have been vasectomized, and almost a half million more undergo this operation every year. Despite careful counseling and warning that this procedure must be considered a permanent step, about 1 percent of these men change their minds at a later date. A common cause for wanting to have the vasectomy reversed is that a marriage has broken up and the man has remarried several years later. In this new marriage both husband and wife generally find themselves wanting to have more children. The death of a child, an improvement in financial stability, or simply a change of heart may result in intense regret at having been sterilized.

One patient of mine was working abroad as a foreign diplomat and only got to visit the United States two weeks of every year. He and his wife had two healthy children and decided that their family was complete. On one of their trips back to the United States to visit their parents, the husband had a vasectomy performed. The day after his vasectomy, his wife was killed in an automobile accident and one child was in critical condition for several weeks. He knew just one day after his vasectomy that it had been a terrible mistake.

Our lives and our families are held together by such thin threads that few of us can feel quite comfortable, at least while we are young, with the decision to be sterilized. A patient of mine from Oregon had two healthy children, a wonderful wife, a beautiful home, and just about everything anyone could want out of life. His third child, a boy, was born on Christmas Day and was an absolute culmination of all their desires. The patient waited several months to make sure the child would be healthy before having his vasectomy performed by his local urologist. One month after the operation he and his wife noticed a lump on the little four-month-old child's arm—which turned out to be a rare and incurable malignant tumor of the muscle. The child died four months later. The couple knew that having another child would not replace the one they lost, but they simply had to have another child. Ironically, this was a couple that had experienced great difficulty in having children in the first place, and when they had all the children they wanted, he had a vasectomy performed. Yet everything seemed to change overnight and they suddenly came to regret their "permanent" decision. Fortunately, we have developed a delicate new microsurgical technique which has substantially improved the outlook for such patients.

## THE MICROSURGICAL OPERATION TO REVERSE VASECTOMY

Though it is easy to perform a vasectomy (it takes only five minutes in the doctor's office), it is very difficult to put it back together because of the microscopic size of the inner canal which carries the sperm (Fig. 17). The outer diameter of the vas deferens is fairly large, about one-eighth of an inch, and the tough outer muscular wall makes it feel like a copper wire through the scrotum. It is certainly an easy structure for the surgeon to identify and cut. But the diameter of the inner canal which carries the sperm is about one-seventieth to one-hundredth of an inch, or roughly the size of a pinpoint. This inner canal has a lining which is about three cells thick, approximately 1/2000 of an inch. Vasectomy had always been considered a relatively permanent condition because of the obvious difficulty in surgically reconnecting such a delicate, tiny tube. With intricate microsurgical techniques, this problem of reconnecting the vas deferens has now essentially been solved.

Very few surgeons are yet able to perform such surgery, however. In order to achieve a nonobstructed reconnection, it is necessary to stitch accurately the delicate inner lining in a leakproof fashion using a thread invisible to the naked eye. The inner canal is only the diameter of a pinpoint. The thicker muscular wall (one-sixteenth of an inch on each side) is then stitched just as precisely to allow proper muscular contraction to milk the sperm into the ejaculate at the time of orgasm. This surgery is all performed under a microscope with very high magnification, using delicate instruments and microscopic thread especially designed for this purpose.

This microsurgical technique is equally successful in cases where previous attempts at vasectomy reversal have failed. In these circumstances the scar tissue from the previous surgery may make the operation somewhat more difficult, but it should not interfere with obtaining an accurate reconnection.

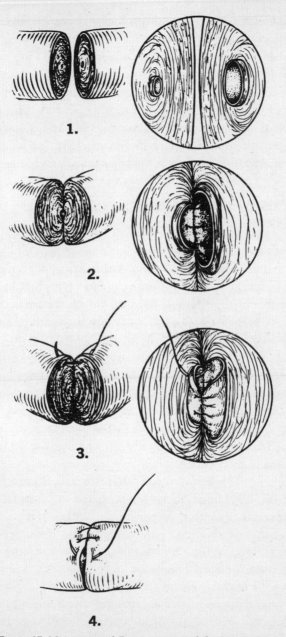

1.

2.

3.

4.

*Figure 17.* Microsurgical Reconnection of the Vas Deferens.

The use of a microscope alone does not ensure that an accurate reconnection will be achieved, however. The surgeon must spend a great deal of time practicing before he develops sufficient skill to do this sort of surgery with confidence. It is important to understand that even with very crude surgical techniques, some sperm can often be found afterward in the ejaculate. But the mere appearance of sperm in the ejaculate does not indicate any likelihood of fertility or subsequent pregnancy. If the amount and quality of sperm is poor, then pregnancy rates will be very low.

## WHAT HAS VASECTOMY DONE TO THE DUCTS OF MY TESTICLES?

After vasectomy, the testicle continues to produce fluid and sperm, which accumulate and expand the entire duct system that normally carries the sperm into the ejaculate. This buildup of pressure is not felt by the patient because the ducts are so tiny that none of these events is noticeable. Luckily the epididymis is capable of reabsorbing a lot of this fluid and serves as a sort of safety valve, blowing off some of the excess pressure before it can do harm. Eventually, however, this safety valve becomes inadequate and pressure builds up to a point where rupture occurs in the epididymis. The testicle itself is never affected by vasectomy; only the ducts that drain it are. Damage created by the pressure in the ducts is what prevents some patients from recovering normal fertility after vasectomy reversal.

The longer the interval of time that has passed since the vasectomy, the less likelihood there is of recovering normal fertility. When a reversal operation is performed within ten years of the original vasectomy, about 90 percent of the patients develop normal sperm counts. When the vasectomy occurred more than ten years before the reversal operation, only about 50 percent of the patients would develop normal sperm counts. However, now we can even repair the ruptured epididymal ducts and thus improve even further the success rate in men whose vasectomy is over ten years old.

Ironically, it is the sloppier vasectomies, the ones that result in sperm leakage at the vasectomy site, that have the best outlook for reversal. This is because these patients have a persistent low-grade leakage of sperm from the cut end of the vas deferens. A small lump, called a sperm granuloma, forms at the cut end of the vas deferens. This lump, which can be felt through the scrotum, is a dynamic structure, with sperm constantly leaking into it and being reabsorbed sufficiently to prevent the pressure increase in the sperm duct that would normally occur. Patients with sperm granulomas have the greatest chance of recovering normal fertility after a vasectomy reversal, regardless of how much time has passed since the vasectomy was performed.

## RECOVERY OF FERTILITY AFTER VASECTOMY REVERSAL

Sperm counts do not return to normal immediately after vasectomy reversal. All of the old sperm which have been stored up over the years since the vasectomy have died of old age, since the lifetime of a sperm after it leaves the testicle and enters the epididymis is less than a month. After the sperm die they slowly deteriorate, the tails breaking off until finally there remain only degenerate-looking sperm heads. This dead sperm material must be cleaned out after the vasectomy is reversed in order to make room for a fresh crop of sperm, which usually does not appear until at least three months later.

Occasionally a very long period of time, even one or two years, is required for complete recovery of adequate sperm motility after vasectomy reversal. This is because the dilated epididymal duct, draining sperm from the testicles into the vas deferens, energizes the sperm so that they will have motility when ejaculated. Until this epididymal duct recovers completely, it cannot adequately energize the sperm. The best treatment for most men with high sperm counts—but poor motility—is time. In many cases the epididymis will recover, but it may take several years.

When the patient has a normal sperm count after vasectomy reversal and the wife is not yet pregnant, it is important that she be evaluated. Several years ago I operated on a history professor to reverse a vasectomy, and one year after the operation he had a perfectly normal sperm count with fifty-five million sperm per cc and 90 percent motility. His wife, however, had not gotten pregnant yet, and his local urologist decided without much thought to put him on hormone therapy. The wife had not been evaluated, but if she had been, they would have discovered (as I did on the telephone) that she had had irregular menstrual bleeding off and on for the last year and a half, and indeed had been placed on birth control pills temporarily by her obstetrician to regulate her periods. So how could she possibly get pregnant?

Another patient of mine, who took quite some time (more than two years) to impregnate his wife after vasectomy reversal, had a much more marginal sperm count and his motility even after one year was still only 10 percent. This patient had had a previous unsuccessful attempt at reconnection of the vas deferens five years earlier, elsewhere. He had had sperm in the ejaculate, but an extremely low count (less than two million per cc) and no motility. For five years he had, understandably, been unsuccessful in impregnating his wife. We reoperated using microsurgical techniques to get an accurate reconnection and bypass the obstructed previous attempt at reconnection. The patient's sperm count went up to forty million rather quickly, but his motility remained low. There were many consultations, during which the patient pressed me for some sort of hormonal therapy to try to improve his motility. During the difficult two years of waiting after our microscopic reoperation, sometimes marked by frustration and anger on the part of the patient and his wife, I came to realize how much easier it is for me to advise a couple to have patience and avoid quacky remedies than it is for the couple simply to sit tight and trust. Finally, after almost two years of waiting, the motility of the husband's sperm rose to 30 percent and his wife became pregnant.

## REOPERATING ON PATIENTS WHO HAVE HAD
## UNSUCCESSFUL ATTEMPTS AT VASECTOMY REVERSAL

Many patients who have had unsuccessful vasectomy reversals are told that they might as well give up, when actually in most of these cases fertility can be restored by a reoperation. One of my patients was a very hard-working Mexican-American from California who was raising three beautiful children, two girls and one boy, holding several jobs, and saving up money to give them a home and the education he never had. Suddenly his boy came down with a rare and incurable illness which baffled his doctors and finally resulted in a deep coma and death. He was beside himself with grief, and decided shortly thereafter to go to one of the nation's leading medical centers and try to reverse the vasectomy that had been performed three years earlier when he had thought his family was complete. The doctors at this medical center explored the patient's scrotum and found no vas deferens whatsoever. Apparently this patient's vasectomy had been performed so radically that there was no vas at all in the scrotal area. His doctor sadly closed the incision, and when the patient woke up he explained to him that there was no hope.

One year later the man chanced to read an article in his local paper written by a former patient of mine. He called the newspaper and talked to the reporter, who suggested the patient should contact me. When I explained to him that the large amount of vas deferens removed should not make any difference in his prospects for recovering fertility, even though it might make for a much larger and more difficult operation, he seemed unable to believe me. He asked for several more opinions, all of which concurred with the medical center where he had had his original surgery, that indeed he didn't have any chance at all, since there was no vas deferens in his scrotum. He finally decided to come to our clinic, anyway, and have another attempt at surgery. We found, as expected, that there was no vas deferens in the scrotum, and our incision had to be extended somewhat into the abdomen. The male is endowed with such an excess length of vas deferens that we were able to free his up, bring it into the scrotum, and very accurately reconnect it under the microscope. The patient now has a normal sperm count, and his wife is now pregnant.

There are countless other patients, with similar stories, who have given up simply because their first efforts at reversal of the vasectomy have failed. Most of the failures of vasectomy reversal are simply caused by an inaccurate reconnection. In a smaller number of cases, permanent damage has already occurred, caused by the pressure buildup after vasectomy. Even that damage now can often be repaired. The only way to know is to reoperate, using very delicate and refined microsurgery.

## Obstruction to Sperm Outflow in Patients Who Have Not Had Vasectomy

When a man's sperm count is zero, and a testicle biopsy shows normal sperm production, there has to be an obstruction somewhere along the duct that conveys sperm to the ejaculate. In some cases the man has actually been born with this obstruction and has never had sperm in his ejaculate. In other cases the obstruction results from an infection which leads to scarring. With modern surgical innovations, the outlook for correcting these obstructions is very good, but the surgery is delicate and intricate.

Prostatitis and other infections of the male genital tract are fairly common in young men. Occasionally an infection will spread down the vas deferens into the epididymis and cause a massive swelling of the scrotum. Often the infection is subtle and the patient does not know he has a problem until he tries to have children. Despite antibiotics and the cure of the infection, the epididymis usually heals with scar tissue and becomes obstructed. Thus an otherwise perfectly fertile man may have total obstruction of sperm outflow.

I had a patient from California who developed exactly this problem after he and his wife had put off having children for several years. He was thirty-eight and she was thirty-one, and they were just about to start trying to have children when the epididymitis suddenly attacked him. The first doctor who saw him when he came in with painful testicles made a misdiagnosis of mumps, and told him just to rest and take warm baths. The epididymis and entire scrotal contents then swelled to enormous proportions (almost the size of a grapefruit on each side), and the patient quite intelligently sought another opinion. The second doctor was a urologist who was a bit more knowledgeable in this field and immediately placed him on the proper antibiotic. The epididymitis went away and the patient appeared to recover normally. However, when the urologist checked his sperm count three months later, fearful of what might have happened, indeed there were no longer any sperm in his ejaculate.

His urologist took the proper next step and admitted him to the hospital for one day to perform a testicle biopsy. This is a very simple operation usually performed under a general anesthetic and requiring about ten minutes, and it is not very painful. Without the biopsy, however, one has no way of knowing whether the absence of sperm is due to a problem with the testicle or to obstruction. In this case the biopsy showed normal sperm production, and the patient was sent to me for microsurgery to repair the intricate duct system that conveys the sperm from the testicle to the vas deferens.

The patient's sperm count one month after the operation showed only a few sperm. The sperm count after two months showed no sperm at all, but we knew that it was too early to expect adequate sperm production. After three months the patient had forty-two million sperm per cc with 50 percent motility, and he has remained in that fertile range ever since the surgery. Before the advent of modern microsurgery, such a patient would have had the worst possible outlook for recovering fertility. Now such a patient has an even better prognosis than those who come in simply with low sperm counts.

Obstruction such as this patient experienced usually occurs in the epididymis. Congenital obstruction may occur in the epididymis, the vas deferens, or the ejaculatory duct close to the prostate gland. The major problem with congenital obstruction is that the epididymis and the entire duct system have been subjected to high pressure for an inordinately long time. Secondary damage may already have occurred. Thus even if the original area of obstruction is fixed, other areas of obstruction caused by leakage and blowouts may have to be fixed also.

Even with modern microsurgical techniques, some patients with congenital obstruction cannot be helped. If they are born with complete absence of the vas deferens, or with an ejaculatory duct obstruction several inches from the prostate, there is no reasonable solution to their problem. The easiest and best course in such cases is artificial donor insemination, which will be discussed in a later chapter. There are some new operations pioneered in Belgium for patients with totally absent vas deferens, whereby a small pouch is created in the scrotum where sperm can accumulate and be aspirated with a hypodermic needle for artificial insemination of the wife. These operations are still experimental and the success rate has been no higher than 10 percent. Thus, while many men with blockage of the ductal system will have to accept the reality of artificial donor insemination, the majority now have an excellent outlook for recovering fertility thanks to fantastic new microsurgical techniques.

## Hormone Treatment to Improve the Sperm Count

Most men with a low sperm count have no obviously treatable cause such as varicocele, previous vasectomy, or obstruction. For years we have looked for some sort of hormonal treatment, similar to inducing ovulation in women, that might improve the sperm count, but the results have frequently been disappointing and the scientific work a bit sloppy. Thus, when a man with a low sperm count goes to see a urologist, he takes the risk of being subjected to a whole barrage of medications, diet, and hormone treatments, which may have significant side effects, but none of which has been clearly proved to increase the sperm count or the chances for pregnancy. This is not a blanket condemnation, but only a warning that any hormone therapy is in a sense experimental. You should therefore be aware of what rational basis there is (if any) for these witchcraftlike therapies.

Just the other day a patient came into the office because of a "low" sperm count (thirty-two million per cc, with 40 percent motility); he had been given thyroid supplements and vitamin E without ever having had a physical examination. When two tablets of thyroid per day didn't do any good, the dose was increased to five thyroid tablets per day. By the time I saw him he was jittery, suffering from insomnia, and he had all of the effects of a highly increased metabolic rate—but no improvement in his sperm count. Not only did this patient have an undiagnosed varicocele which could have been treated if he had undergone a proper physical examination, but in addition it was clear upon subsequent evaluation of his wife that despite having regular menstrual periods, she was not ovulating. If this patient had had an opportunity to read the following sections, he might have considered more carefully whether to submit himself to such questionable but widely available therapy.

## THE FERTILE EUNUCH

There is a rare condition known as the fertile-eunuch syndrome which lends many clues about what sort of hormone treatment might conceivably affect sperm production in men with low sperm counts. Fertile eunuchs are men who are born with normal-sized testicles which have active sperm production, but which have very few of the Leydig cells which make the male hormone testosterone. These men are essentially eunuchs, with no sexual development, little body hair, and a tiny penis; yet they produce sperm. If administered HCG (human chorionic gonadotropin), their testicles suddenly begin to produce male hormone, they go through puberty, and they become normal men. Their sperm counts before treatment are very low, but after treatment the counts come up to normal.

This bizarre syndrome demonstrates that sperm production can take place in the absence of male hormone although such sperm are inadequate in number and quality for impregnation. When administered HCG, which stimulates the testicles to make their own testosterone, these men become fertile.

The fact that the fertile eunuch is not truly fertile until his hormone deficiency is eliminated gives us some clues about what might be expected from hormone therapy in the more common situation where an otherwise normal man has a low sperm count. Some such patients may possibly respond to hormone therapy as do fertile eunuchs.

### CLOMID (CLOMIPHENE CITRATE)

Clomid, which is very effective in stimulating women to ovulate, also may improve the fertility of some men. It works in both sexes by stimulating the primitive region of the brain to cause the pituitary gland to release the hormones FSH and LH. In men, FSH and LH work hand-in-hand to stimulate sperm production. While LH stimulates the Leydig cells to produce testosterone, FSH stimulates the cells that line the sperm-producing tubules to pull testosterone into the tubules. Unless sufficient testosterone gets into the tubules, sperm production is deficient. Clomid is thus commonly given to infertile men with low sperm counts in the hopes of increasing their fertility by raising both FSH and LH levels.

It appears to be a very safe drug, having been used for many years in women quite successfully. In a few experiments it has been found to produce visual disturbances when administered in enormously high doses, so caution is required for those who have eyesight problems. Though Clomid appears to be safe, it has not yet been approved officially by the FDA for use in men except on an experimental basis, but it is commonly available if the patient gives informed consent to its use.

Studies that have purported to show that Clomid causes great improvement in the majority of men have, in most cases, been performed very poorly. Very few sperm counts were performed on each patient in these optimistic studies, and the modest improvements that were found may have been no more than random variations in the sperm counts. Any hope that Clomid will be a cure-all for male infertility is misplaced. The drug only helps a few. Many urologists prescribe Clomid casually, and have no idea whether it has truly improved the fertility of their patients.

The only carefully controlled study of the effects of Clomid on infertile men was performed at Cardiff University in Great Britain. One hundred and fourteen infertile men with low sperm counts were given either Clomid or a placebo (a sugar pill designed to look like the Clomid pill), and neither the doctor nor the patient knew which patients received Clomid and which the placebo. As a whole, the group taking Clomid showed no striking improvement compared to the group not taking Clomid. Nonetheless, Clomid does produce a striking improvement in a small number of men. If we could determine ahead of time which patients might benefit from this therapy, we could prevent a great deal of anguish resulting from false hopes.

One side effect of Clomid in males is that the dramatic increase in testosterone frequently stirs up the libido considerably, so that sex may take place much more often. In females Clomid has no such effect, because in women the increased FSH and LH do not affect testosterone production.

### HCG (HUMAN CHORIONIC GONADOTROPIN)

There has been a great deal of talk about routine use of the hormone HCG in men with low sperm counts to improve their fertility. This is perhaps one of the hormones most commonly administered to men with low sperm counts, but there is very little we can say about it since little has been published in the scientific literature. One thing is certain, however: three injections of this hormone every week for three months is rather uncomfortable. It would be worth the discomfort if the patient had some way of knowing ahead of time whether he might be one of the few who would respond. Although this hormone can quite dramatically improve sperm production in rare individuals, such as the fertile eunuch, it should not be given without a thorough evaluation including many sperm counts, testicle biopsy, and hormone determinations.

Essentially the only carefully controlled study on HCG given to infertile men was performed by Dr. Richard Sherins, the head of the reproduction research branch of the National Institutes of Health in Bethesda, Maryland. Dr. Sherins emphasizes that sperm counts vary greatly from month to month, and certainly during any three-month cycle the man who appeared to have a low sperm count may suddenly come up to normal, simply because his general condition or a chronic infection may have improved. No patient was admitted to Dr. Sherins's treatment program unless sperm counts had been performed every two weeks for six months and a consistent and repeatable average determined. Only this way would it be possible to tell whether any change in the sperm count was due to therapy or simply to normal variation. Dr. Sherins demonstrated that HCG resulted in no increase at all in the sperm count and resulted in no pregnancies. In fact, sperm counts decreased in several cases. When Dr. Sherins reevaluated the wives of all these patients, he found that a significant number had subtle gynecological problems, and at least half of these "normal" wives became pregnant when they were properly treated.

## PERGONAL

Pergonal, the commercial preparation of the hormone FSH, is extraordinarily effective in inducing ovulation in women who do not ovulate. If any hormonal treatment would seem capable of raising the infertile man's sperm count, it would likely be Pergonal. Unfortunately, there have been very few studies on treatment of infertile men with Pergonal, probably because it is so expensive.

One use of Pergonal in males involves patients who have had their pituitary glands removed in neurosurgery. In such cases, production of FSH and LH ceases, and the men quickly become sterile eunuchs. Since FSH and LH are both necessary for adequate sperm production, the ideal replacement is to administer both of these hormones. However, FSH is so terribly expensive that it could never be administered on a long-term basis. Such patients therefore usually receive HCG injections simply to maintain testosterone production and male characteristics. Without FSH, they continue to have sperm production, but it is generally inadequate. As soon as they decide they want to have children, the administration of Pergonal (FSH) increases their sperm count dramatically, and makes them fertile so that they can impregnate their wives. When the FSH is discontinued, and only HCG administered to maintain their maleness, the sperm counts again go down to much lower, inadequate levels.

When used in the more common situation of the infertile man with a normal pituitary, the sperm-producing effect of FSH is not this dramatic. Pergonal has been reported to increase the sperm count in a few patients. However, there is no clear evidence that the improvement in sperm count that occasionally occurs is caused by the drug rather than just by spontaneous variation. Again the only good studies available were directed by Dr. Sherins at the National Institutes of Health. Unfortunately, in the patients that he has thus far reported on, even Pergonal, the most expensive and the most powerful drug available for stimulating fertility in either men or women, had very little effect on sperm counts, and no pregnancies resulted.

However, we should not be too depressed by these early results. There may be small groups of patients with low sperm counts who will respond to specific hormone stimulation. We do not know yet whether this powerful drug Pergonal is going to have major benefits for some men with low sperm counts. But at least with the type of careful study being performed at centers such as the National Institutes of Health, we should soon find the answer.

GONADOTROPIN-RELEASING HORMONE (GNRH)

GNRH is the hormone released from the primitive region of the brain, the hypothalamus, that sets the whole sexual hormone apparatus in motion. Since its discovery in 1971 there has been some hope that administration of this hormone, or perhaps of synthetic imitations of it, might stimulate the testicles to increase sperm production. Unfortunately, several studies performed by Andrew Schally, the Nobel Prize–winning scientist who discovered this hormone, have thus far failed to demonstrate any improvement in sperm counts.

OTHER "MAGIC POTIONS"

I have had patients referred to me from all over the country who have been given every treatment imaginable, with little rational basis. They have been placed on thyroid medications despite having no thyroid problems. They have been placed on high doses of vitamin E and on low doses of vitamin E. They have been given extra vitamin C; they have been placed on high- and on low-carbohydrate diets, on high-protein and low-protein diets. They have been given testosterone injections, which are actually more effective as contraceptives than as fertility-promoting agents. They have been told to avoid alcohol, smoking, and all of the other bad habits that they probably should be avoiding anyway. None of these therapies has demonstrated any benefit whatsoever in improving male fertility. In view of our obvious state of frustration in dealing with the difficult problem of low sperm counts, physicians have resorted to every possible form of witchcraft, hoping that by accident something useful may be discovered. Often it appears that the patient's mental well-being itself depends on his obtaining some sort of therapy, even if it is just a sugar pill.

The therapies we have discussed in this section may turn out to be effective in certain men. But at this time any hormonal treatment program for a low sperm count is experimental. If a man understands this, and if his doctor is following an orderly, disciplined approach to treatment, then he will be receiving the best that medicine can presently give, and we can only hope that it results in a pregnancy. It is important to remember, though, that at this time the most successful way to overcome a husband's low sperm count is to treat the wife in order to maximize her fertility.

## Saving It Up, Concentration of Sperm for Artificial Insemination, and General Remedies

More important than the total number of sperm in the ejaculate is their concentration. If you are ejaculating a small number of sperm in too large a volume, most of the spermatozoa will not have an opportunity to invade your wife's cervical mucus. The sperm which are present are too diluted to represent a formidable invasion force for the cervix. Therefore if you have a large-volume ejaculate with a relatively low sperm count per cc, your concentration of sperm might be increased by reducing the amount of fluid you ejaculate.

Fortunately in most men the majority of sperm comes out in the first few squirts, and all the rest of the ejaculate harbors little sperm. If the first small portion of your ejaculate is squirted into one jar, and the remainder into a second jar, most of the sperm should be heavily concentrated in the first jar. This is the so-called "split ejaculate." In men who have relatively large ejaculates, with a low concentration of sperm, this method of "split ejaculation" may be very beneficial by increasing the sperm concentration.

There are two ways of utilizing the "split ejaculate." One is simply to "pull out" early—just at the very beginning of ejaculation. This way only the portion of the ejaculate which has the most sperm has gotten in and has not been diluted by the remainder. Another approach is to provide a "split ejaculate" in two separate jars. A gynecologist then checks which specimen has the highest sperm concentration (the first specimen will have the highest concentration in 90 percent of cases), and then artificially inseminates the woman at exactly the right time in her cycle with that concentrated specimen. This way, what few sperm a man does make will have the greatest chance of partaking in that massive armylike invasion of the cervical mucus which requires so many sperm in order for just one to reach the egg.

Sometimes a man may have the opposite problem. He may have a very small ejaculate (less than one-fifth of a teaspoon)—but with a very high concentration of sperm in it. In this case that little bit of ejaculate which has so much sperm in it may not ever make contact with the wife's cervix, but become lost in the vast cavern of the vagina. In addition, patients with too small an ejaculate may not have enough alkalinity to neutralize the acidity of the wife's vagina. The sperm simply will not make it in an acid environment and require a reasonable amount of ejaculate to protect them until they gain access to the cervix. The solution in such cases is to have a gynecologist place the ejaculate right next to the woman's cervix at the most fertile time in her cycle, making sure that the bull's-eye is hit.

One of the most popularly talked-about ideas for improving the man's sperm count is to take multiple ejaculates and freeze them in liquid nitrogen, saving up until enough has been stored to be thawed and pooled for artificial insemination of the wife. The problem with this approach is that in men with very low sperm counts, the only ones who might conceivably benefit from such a procedure, the freezing process is very harmful and an adequately motile sperm count is never achieved.

Even if it were theoretically possible to save it all up this way, just think of the logistics involved. If you had a sperm count of, say, five million sperm per cc with 15 percent motile, and you had the sperm frozen, at least half of those sperm would die from the freezing process; this would leave you no more than 7 percent of five million sperm, or only 0.35 million sperm with any activity at all. It would take approximately one hundred such ejaculations with subsequent storage to provide you with a total of thirty-five million motile sperm. It would be very difficult to find any husband who would be willing to donate one hundred of the perhaps two hundred orgasms he is going to have during the entire year to this process. But even if he were willing, unfortunately such an approach doesn't work because most of the sperm in such poor semen samples are destroyed by the freezing process. Weak sperm simply do not freeze as well as healthy sperm.

Saving up sperm by abstaining from sex is also not as helpful to men with low sperm counts as it might seem to be. Any benefit from saving up all the sperm until the day before ovulation is overshadowed by the higher number of nonmotile and stale sperm that come out after that long a period of abstinence. It is true that the sperm count is markedly diminished in most men the day after an ejaculation, but usually two or three days are quite sufficient for the buildup of maximum sperm count. Intercourse every other day or every third day (whatever is the couple's particular pleasure) is the best approach.

Furthermore, the anxiety and stress that scheduled intercourse places on a relationship can easily disrupt the hypothalamus sufficiently to interfere with the wife's ovulation. When the stress and aggravation created by overattention to the precise timing of intercourse is removed, she may very well then start to ovulate normally again.

Finally, we should always remember the effect that general health and freedom from mental anxiety can have on fertility. While there is a definite relationship between nervous anxiety and infertility in women, in men the effects of stress and anxiety are not as clear. We know that prisoners in Nazi concentration camps during the Holocaust were generally noted to have severely low sperm counts, induced simply by the stress and the poor conditions of their imprisonment. Released from the prison camps to a more normal life, most of them could recover fertility. So in treating the male with a low sperm count, we can't underestimate the importance of time, patience, and gaining an intelligent understanding of what fertility is all about. In fact, that is the reason for this book.

Certainly a fever from a severe flu or generalized infection can result in a very badly depressed sperm count which can last for three months. Recovery from this infection can result in a spectacular improvement in sperm count. Perhaps one of the most effective remedies for men with low sperm counts is to send them to the dentist to make sure there is no hidden abscess somewhere. We have seen quite a few men whose low sperm counts dramatically improved after having a neglected dental problem corrected. Any elevation in temperature to fever levels will result in a prompt depression of sperm production. Sometimes just time and patience will result in an improvement of the sperm count without any treatment at all.

In a small number of infertile men, the problem is simply that the ejaculate is going backward into the bladder and not forward out of the penis. This most commonly occurs in diabetic patients who are otherwise healthy and lead a normal sex life, but have a complication called retrograde ejaculation which occurs from a deterioration in certain nerves caused by the diabetes. These patients are potentially fertile and their orgasms even feel completely normal; their only problem is that the sperm do not come out in their ejaculate during intercourse but instead come out in their urine later. Recently we have found that giving these patients simple cold tablets, like Ornade (which normally shrinks the swollen tissue of the nose to make the cold-sufferer more comfortable), is also effective in closing the internal sphincter, and allowing these patients to ejaculate sperm out of their penis rather than backward into the bladder. Such patients then have no difficulty in impregnating their wives. There is a rational, logical basis to this treatment, and it has worked repeatedly in carefully disciplined scientific studies. Nonetheless, the fact that a common cold remedy can convert some absolutely sterile men to complete fertility in less than a month must make us all a little slow to condemn the seemingly irrational approach of some doctors who may subject their patients to all kinds of equally apparently crazy remedies in the hope of improving the sperm count.

# ·6·

# Artificial Insemination and Sperm-Banking

## Artificial Insemination by Donor

### WHOSE BABY IS IT?

Ten years ago, when a couple reached a dead end in their quest to have a baby, the solution would have been to adopt. Society was burdened with a relatively large supply of unwanted children. Since the popularization of abortion and of a wide variety of birth control measures, there are now very few babies available for adoption, and the wait for those couples who are successful is often more than five years. The solution today for couples who are unable to adopt a child (when the wife's infertility problem can be treated but the husband's cannot) is simply to "adopt sperm." Since unwanted babies are no longer easily available, the only choice in a sense is to adopt the baby at a much earlier stage, i.e., prior to conception. Artificial insemination, using the sperm of an anonymous donor, is now the most popular and realistic solution for couples in which the husband's infertility cannot be cured.

From a medical point of view artificial insemination is extraordinarily simple. It was first successfully used in women by the famous physician John Hunter in England in the eighteenth century. A sperm specimen obtained from the donor through masturbation is drawn up into a syringe, and then simply squirted into the vagina near the cervix. Since the sperm are only capable of fertilization for twenty-four to forty-eight hours in the female reproductive tract, and since the egg is only capable of being fertilized within eight hours of ovulation, the insemination must be timed appropriately just before ovulation.

Artificial insemination was first successfully performed in the United States in 1866 by Dr. Marion Sims, but the sperm used was almost exclusively that of the husband. Later, in 1890, Dr. Robert Dickinson of New York started using artificial insemination with donor sperm when the husband had untreatable infertility. This early use of artificial insemination by donor was carried out in great secrecy. However, it has now become so popular that more than ten thousand babies are born every year in the United States as a result of it. Patients are accepting it when there is no other solution, and many of the psychological, social, and legal fears about it are beginning to disappear.

Georgia, in 1964, was the first state to issue legislation that guarantees that a child conceived in this manner will be considered legitimate. Oklahoma passed a similar law in 1967, and Kansas in 1968. Even prior to these legislative decrees, common law provided some protection for the legitimacy of such children. Unless it is proved that the husband had no access to the wife, any child born of her is considered to be his by the law. Whether or not the husband is the true father, he is the legal father of any child born to his wife while they are living together.

I recently saw a patient who had had a vasectomy performed in 1974, thinking he would not want to have children. Later, he and his wife changed their views and became very anxious to have a family. He had two attempts at vasectomy reversal elsewhere, which failed to restore any sperm to his ejaculate. Subsequently his wife underwent artificial insemination with semen from an anonymous donor and she became pregnant. They had a beautiful little baby by artificial insemination. She was three months old when the patient was first referred to me. I felt that by using microsurgical techniques we could restore his fertility, but wished first to explore his feelings about the daughter he already had. The patient clearly loved her very much from the minute that she was born, and if this surgery was not successful, he was perfectly ready to have another child by artificial insemination. The patient did not feel that the genetic contribution was as important as his devotion to the child, and so we performed a reversal operation. The patient regained a normal sperm count, and impregnated his wife one year later. They now have two children and love them equally.

Prior to the wife's undergoing artificial insemination, the doctor will always have both wife and husband sign a special consent form which states: (1) that any children produced by artificial insemination will be their own legitimate children and their heirs; (2) that they waive forever any right to disclaim such a child as their own; and (3) that the nature of the agreement will make it confidential among the husband, the wife, and the doctor. The agreement will state that the husband and wife rely upon the judgment and discretion of the doctor to choose a donor whose physical and mental characteristics are compatible with those of the husband. They then must agree that they understand the doctor cannot be held responsible for any physical or mental characteristics of any child so produced. At the moment of conception the husband must automatically accept the child as his own.

Frequently the husband has a very low sperm count, one which would have a very small chance of ever resulting in conception, but at least there are a few sperm present. Such a patient can never be sure that a child conceived while his wife undergoes artificial insemination is not a product of his sperm. The wife is often told to have intercourse with her husband shortly after artificial donor insemination. There is a scientific as well as a psychological reason for this. Sperm enter the cervical mucus two abreast and form lines of attack along the border between the semen and the cervical mucus. The first sperm to get in frequently die as they carve a path through the cervical mucus. Then others move in along the same path. It seems that there is a process of sacrifice and waste whereby the earliest sperm to overcome the barrier of the cervical mucus die while establishing a portal for other sperm to enter.  A large number of good sperm may have to be around in order to create a path into the cervical mucus for others to follow. There is always the possibility, however slight, that a sperm of the husband's may very well be the one finally to fertilize the egg.


HOW IS IT DONE?

The woman's ovulatory pattern as determined by basal body temperature charts, cervical mucus production, and dilatation of the cervix are required to pinpoint the time of ovulation so that the sperm can be introduced on the best day.  However, sometimes the precise timing of ovulation becomes impossible, because the emotional stress placed upon the wife affects her hypothalamus to the extent that she may ovulate late, or she may even fail to ovulate. For this reason the bedside manner of the physician is very important.  If the wife is terrified by an inadequate understanding of what is being done, she may very easily stop ovulating altogether. In such cases, ironically, when the program of artificial insemination is abandoned, her periods often return to normal and she begins to ovulate again.

Because of the difficulty of pinpointing the exact time of ovulation under the psychological stress of artificial insemination, the physician may place the wife on Clomid or HCG, to induce regular ovulation.  Women treated with Clomid tend to ovulate right at mid-cycle, around day fourteen or fifteen, despite the emotional stress that might otherwise interfere with their cycles.  The patient is placed on one Clomid tablet each day for five days beginning on the fifth day of her cycle.  Then about five days after completion of the Clomid treatment, usually day fourteen of her cycle, artificial insemination is performed.  Using this approach, a number of doctors have reported a higher pregnancy rate within a fewer number of cycles than when the time of ovulation is not artificially controlled.

Regardless of whether ovulation is induced with drugs or allowed to proceed spontaneously, the woman must continue to take her basal body temperature.  The doctor will inseminate her on what he thinks is the day before ovulation, and again two days later if her temperature has not risen one day after the first insemination. Since the sperm are only able to fertilize the egg for a period of forty-eight hours, if the temperature does not rise one day after the first insemination, she will be inseminated again with the hope that even though she is ovulating somewhat later than expected, the second insemination may allow her to conceive.

The actual technique of artificial insemination is simple and entirely painless. The patient is placed in position as for a routine pelvic exam and the vaginal speculum is inserted just as though she were having a Pap smear. The donor's semen is then either squirted against the cervix into the recesses of the vagina, or placed in a plastic-type cap which is then put over the cervix and allowed to stay in position for a half hour to three hours. Whichever method is used, the patient is usually requested to remain in position for one half hour, allowing plenty of time for the sperm to gain access to the cervical mucus. After that first half hour most of the sperm that would have any chance of reaching the egg will have already entered, and the patient is then allowed to leave. Insemination is only performed if the woman's cervix opening is dilated and if she is producing abundant cervical mucus, indicating that she is about to ovulate. If her cervix is not yet "ripe," the physician may ask her to return one or two days later. If on the other hand her cervix appears "ripe," and she undergoes insemination but her temperature does not go up, she will have to be inseminated again in two days.

DONOR SELECTION

Selection of an appropriate donor is probably the physician's heaviest responsibility in artificial insemination. Obviously the donor has to be of excellent physical and mental stock, with proven fertility. Skin, hair, and eye color should match the patient's husband as closely as possible, and their blood types should be compatible. The donor is asked to abstain from intercourse for two days, and then masturbate into a clean container. A tiny portion of this specimen is examined microscopically to make sure that he has a good sperm sample, and to make sure there are no bacteria such as gonorrhea in the specimen. The remainder is used for the insemination.

The donor must always be anonymous. Occasionally the couple may request a particular donor, but many problems exist when the biological father is known to the couple. In actuality most donors turn out to be medical students or interns who are healthy and readily available in the medical community. Donors are paid for their services. Just as their identity is never revealed to the couple, the couple's identity is never revealed to the donor.

## PREGNANCY RATES WITH ARTIFICIAL INSEMINATION

In most artificial insemination clinics, 90 percent of the women who eventually get pregnant do so within the first six months. This has led to the erroneous notion that if the woman is not pregnant within six months it might be wise for her to give up, since she is not likely to become pregnant with future inseminations. Patients are frequently warned that 80 percent will achieve pregnancy within one year, but very few pregnancies will occur after that. Because the majority of women become pregnant relatively soon, and the percentage of women who achieve pregnancy after six months is relatively small, many patients who are fertile (and who should have a normal 20 percent expectation of pregnancy with each insemination) are erroneously told that they might as well just give up, and not to go through the frustration of more failures. A simple review of the statistics presented in Chapter 3 lends a more optimistic outlook. Pregnancy rates with artificial insemination are as good as normally occurring pregnancy rates in an otherwise fertile population.

## Frozen Sperm and Sperm Banks

All men dream from time to time about the possibility of immortality. Science-fiction novelists frequently toy with the idea of human beings being placed in a deep freeze just prior to the moment of death, to be revived perhaps two hundred years later, at which time science may have better treatments for illnesses and a way of prolonging life indefinitely. Life is in a sense a series of chemical events proceeding irreversibly toward death, and these chemical events cannot take place at −400°. Thus if an organism can be placed in a deep freeze, it could be preserved until a future century, and revived with subsequent warming.

Of course, freezing large animals would kill them immediately because of damage created by crystallization of water within their cells during the freezing process. However, it has been known since 1776 that human sperm are remarkably resistant to the damaging effects of freezing. In that year an Italian scientist exposed spermatozoa to freezing temperatures and noted that after warming, some of them regained their motility. A full ninety years later another Italian scientist again demonstrated that human sperm can be frozen and survive thawing, and he speculated that in the future (remember, this was in 1866) frozen semen might be used not only in breeding the finest farm animals, but for saving the sperm of a man going off to war so that his wife might have a legitimate child from him even though he died on the battlefield.

Although these relatively crude early studies established that sperm could survive freezing and thawing, the number of sperm surviving was so small (fewer than 10 percent) that there was no possibility of practical application. But in 1949 British scientists discovered completely by accident that if a relatively common chemical, glycerol, is added to the semen before it is frozen, the majority of the sperm survive freezing and thawing uneventfully. The researchers who made this discovery were so surprised to find live, healthy sperm in large concentrations after thawing that they had to go back to their laboratory shelf to find out which of the chemicals accidentally added to their sperm suspension was the one that protected the sperm against freezing. They finally discovered that it was glycerol. It took very little time after their remarkable discovery in 1949 for frozen-sperm banks to rapidly find acceptance in the field of cattle breeding, and today the vast majority of calves born in the world are the result of artificial insemination from frozen bull semen.

In 1953, four years after this discovery, it was demonstrated that frozen and thawed human sperm could result in pregnancy and the delivery of normal babies. The first human-sperm bank was established in 1954. Doctors originally thought that, using this method of freezing sperm, a husband with a very low sperm count could have as many as fifty ejaculates frozen and stored for use in artificial insemination of the wife; they hoped that with such a large number of sperm, the wife would be more likely to get pregnant. These hopes were dashed by the discovery that sperm from infertile men tolerate the freezing process very poorly. There is so much sperm death caused by freezing, even with glycerol, that a decent specimen could never be obtained for inseminating the wife. Doctors have since come to understand that some men's sperm tolerates freezing better than others. Even men whose sperm usually would freeze well have variations from ejaculate to ejaculate. Sometimes their ejaculates freeze and thaw without any significant loss, and at other times they freeze and thaw very poorly.

The technique for freezing and storing the sperm is extremely simple. A fresh semen specimen is collected in a sterile container, and several drops of glycerol, equal to one-tenth of the volume of the specimen, are added to the jar. This mixture is then drawn up into a straw. The specimen is held over the vapors of liquid nitrogen to freeze it, and it is then inserted into the liquid nitrogen bath for permanent storage. When the time comes to thaw the frozen sperm, the plastic straw is simply removed from the liquid nitrogen bath, and either placed in warm water for one minute or left on a table at room temperature to thaw.

Although some doctors report no loss of viability of sperm for a period of at least ten years in liquid nitrogen, others have demonstrated a definite though slow loss of fertility in an increasing percentage of the samples after three years of storage. If the patient's sperm tolerate a rapid freeze-thaw test well, then most of his samples, though not all of them, are likely to survive well for at least three years in liquid nitrogen. There have been births of normal children from sperm that have been stored over ten years, but this is the exception rather than the rule.

Fertility is lower with frozen than with fresh semen specimens. Yet if only the best donors are used for freezing, the fertility of that semen is not significantly impaired by the freezing and thawing process. Even though a specimen might start out with 80 percent motility, and after thawing two years later have only 40 percent motility, this does not have a dramatic effect on the ability of that sample to fertilize and result in conception. Furthermore, the children born of such conceptions are perfectly normal. In fact all of the studies on artificial insemination using frozen sperm have demonstrated a lower incidence of abnormal children than one would encounter in a normal population. Apparently genes are not harmed by the freeze-thaw procedure. Whatever harm may come to sperm, in structure or in ability to fertilize, there does not appear to be any increased risk of defective children. Extensive experience both in cattle and in humans has now documented that artificial insemination with frozen sperm from sperm banks is safe. Literally thousands of pregnancies and births in humans from this technique have been reported in the scientific literature.

The major benefit of sperm-banking at the present stage of our knowledge is to create easier and more convenient programs of artificial insemination in cases where the husband's infertility is not treatable. The ability of sperm freezing to preserve our genes indefinitely, for use at a future date, is presently limited to the few lucky individuals whose sperm freezes and stores consistently well, but it will not work for most ordinary men.

## Artificial Insemination of the Husband's Sperm

Many doctors have tried to increase the chances of pregnancy in a woman whose husband has a very low sperm count by placing his semen directly on her cervix. Unfortunately, many studies by doctors around the country have shown that, except in certain special cases, this approach is no better than natural intercourse for getting the wife pregnant, and certainly is less enjoyable.

Of the sperm deposited in the vagina, 99.9 percent never

reach the uterus. Normally, of the millions of spermatozoa that are deposited in the vagina during coitus only a few thousand ever get into the uterine cavity. Therefore, a number of gynecologists have attempted to solve the problem of low sperm counts by introducing the sperm directly into the wife's uterus, eliminating the wasteful invasion of the cervical mucus. Doctors experimenting in Northern Ireland have reported a 38 percent pregnancy rate in wives of men with sperm counts under ten million sperm per cc. In a limited test, American researchers have achieved pregnancy in five out of nine women with this technique.

This approach is potentially dangerous. Only a small volume of semen can be instilled into the uterus safely. If the entire ejaculate were to be instilled into the uterus, it would cause severe cramps and a very painful reaction. It may be that certain chemicals in the semen are very irritative to the uterus, since injection of so-called "radiopaque dyes" to perform an X ray of the woman's tubes via the uterus does not produce this kind of reaction. Despite these difficulties, the idea of instilling sperm directly into the uterus to overcome the cervical barrier, though experimental and seldom practiced, sounds like an attractive concept.

Instillation of the husband's sperm on the cervix, though usually of little benefit, in a few very special situations is dramatically effective. If the husband has a normal number of sperm with good motility, but the volume of his ejaculate is very low, he may be missing the cervix when he ejaculates. For example, the normal ejaculate has a volume of fluid anywhere from half a teaspoon to one and a half teaspoons. This is sufficient to cover the cervix so that the sperm have an excellent chance of penetrating the mucus. However, some men have a tiny ejaculate volume—as little as one-tenth of a teaspoon. Such a small amount of fluid may harbor an enormous amount of sperm but the sperm have very little chance of reaching the cervical mucus because they are not very likely to get deposited in the right place. Another problem with having a low ejaculate volume is that the sperm become immobilized rather quickly because there is an insufficient amount of semen alkalinity to neutralize the vaginal acid. This problem can be solved by the physician taking the husband's ejaculate and placing it right next to the cervical mucus. In these special cases artificial insemination with the husband's sperm has been very successful.

Another possible benefit of artificial insemination with the husband's sperm is that in the future we may be able to predetermine the baby's sex. The chromosomes that determine whether the child will be female or male are the X and Y sex chromosomes. All eggs have an X chromosome, while half of the sperm have an X chromosome and half have a Y chromosome. The sperm with a Y chromosome will make a boy and those with an X will make a girl. Since every egg has only X chromosomes, it is the sperm type (X or Y) which determines the sex of the baby. (After we had our third son—and no daughters—my little six-year-old David, who had preferred to have a sister, complained to me: "Daddy, don't you have any X sperm at all?")

Countless efforts have been made by a number of researchers to separate X sperm from Y sperm with the hope that, through artificial insemination of the separated portion of the ejaculate, couples would be able to choose the sex of their baby. Although it is possible for us to distinguish under the microscope which sperm are X-bearing and which are Y-bearing, it has not yet been possible to separate them and, therefore, have any influence on the likelihood of the baby's being a boy or a girl. Another intriguing idea which has captured the imagination of many couples is that by delaying intercourse and thus increasing the acidity of the vagina they might in some way be able to influence whether the X sperm or the Y sperm is more likely to fertilize the egg.

Unfortunately, neither of these techniques has yet been very effective.

## Artificial Breeding Techniques in Animals

In dairy cattle the economic advantages of artificial insemination compared with natural mating are enormous. By using frozen semen from the very finest bulls, whose single ejaculate, after thawing, carries a sufficient number of sperm to inseminate a thousand cows, cattlemen have been able to produce prize calves every time with little effort. More than 70 percent of the calves born today are the result of artificial insemination. This explosion in cattle breeding took place after 1949 when the secret of preserving frozen sperm with glycerol was discovered.

In cattle the conception rate obtained with frozen and thawed semen from prize bulls is equivalent to that of fresh semen. Many samples from prize bulls have been preserved satisfactorily for more than twenty years, long after the animals themselves had died. Whereas a good human ejaculate may contain 200 million sperm, the average ejaculate of a bull carries ten billion sperm. In other farm animals, such as sheep and pigs, frozen-thawed sperm has generally been much less fertile than fresh sperm and the applications of sperm-banking for these animals have therefore been very limited.

Although the abundance of sperm in a bull ejaculate would seem quite enough, there have been efforts to increase the sperm concentration in prize bulls even further by giving them hormones in order to increase sperm production. Giving these hormones to cows will certainly cause production of more eggs, but in bulls the administration of these hormones does not have any effect on sperm production. This again underlines the difficulty of improving the sperm count in males by hormonal stimulation.

In cows a small amount of semen can be deposited directly into the uterus, bypassing the cervix. Thus the large waste of sperm involved in the process of cervical mucus invasion (as in humans) is avoided. In sheep the cervix is constricted and folded, so the semen must be deposited right on the surface of the cervix, as in humans. Artificial insemination of pigs is also difficult. The volume of the boar's ejaculate is a full pint, and he inseminates this enormous volume of fluid directly into the sow's uterus by inserting his penis into her cervical opening. This is accomplished by screw-type ridges on the boar's penis which interlock with screw-type grooves in the sow's cervix. Thus a difficult maneuver involving a special rubber tube with a corkscrew tip would be needed to inseminate semen directly into the sow's uterus. Because of such difficulties in most animals, the greatest success with artificial insemination has been with humans and cattle.

The optimum time for insemination is about ten to twelve hours before ovulation. If the animals were allowed to mate normally, of course, they would automatically copulate at the right time, unlike humans. When artificial insemination is being used, however, it is necessary to determine exactly when heat occurs, just prior to ovulation.

## POTENTIAL APPLICATIONS IN HUMANS

Recent success with the introduction of frozen and thawed boar's semen directly into the sow's fallopian tubes gives us some hope that such techniques may be worthwhile in humans where the male has a low sperm count. If thawed boar's semen is inseminated into the sow's reproductive tract in the normal manner, through the cervix, very few eggs are fertilized. On the other hand, if the semen is introduced directly into the oviduct of the sow by surgical techniques, a very high proportion of eggs are fertilized. The major obstacle to successful fertilization with frozen-thawed semen in a pig then appears to be a difficulty with transport of the sperm through the uterus. Conceivably a similar introduction of otherwise relatively infertile human sperm directly into the uterus or the fallopian tubes might lead to a higher pregnancy rate for wives of men with very low sperm counts.

It is not just sperm that we can preserve by freezing. Embryos up to eight days after conception, including mice, rabbits, sheep, and cattle, have been preserved for long periods of time, shipped halfway across the world, reimplanted in females of that species on the other side of the world, and normal babies have thus been born. Although many of these embryos do not survive the freezing and thawing process, a sufficient number grow up into normal, healthy young. In the future, low-temperature preservation not just of sperm, but also of animals in their earliest stages of development, may become widespread. When this becomes possible on a larger scale, not only will prime bulls be able to father literally millions of cattle all around the world, but prize cows will be able to donate all of their eggs to less valuable cows who would then be able to carry those pregnancies all the way to term. These advanced techniques of animal husbandry have been with us for more than a quarter of a century. The same techniques we have developed in these farm animals may in the future help humans who are presently not able to have their own babies.

# ·7·

# Test-Tube Babies and Cloning

## The First Human Test-Tube Baby

On a Tuesday evening, July 25, 1978, at 11:47 P.M., Louise Brown was born, a beautiful, normal, five-pound, twelve-ounce girl with blond hair and blue eyes—the world's first human test-tube baby. Dr. Robert Edwards and Dr. Patrick Steptoe, in a drowsy little clinic near Manchester, England, were responsible for this giant step forward into the "brave new world." Dr. Edwards's first statement upon seeing the child was "The last time I saw the baby it was just eight cells in a test tube. It was beautiful then and it is still beautiful now." The child's mother, Leslie Brown, and father, John Brown, are ordinary working people. They had been married for nine years and were unable to have children. The problem was that the wife's tubes were so badly destroyed by scars and inflammation that even modern microsurgery could not help her. Her ovaries and her uterus were normal, however, and all that was required to grant her dream was to take an egg from her ovary, mix it with her husband's sperm in a test tube, and then reimplant the two-day-old embryo into her womb to grow for the next nine months into a full-term baby.

This achievement was the culmination of twelve years of painstaking research by the two doctors, research which was obviously greeted with a great deal of controversy. Thanks to Drs. Steptoe and Edwards, there is now hope in many otherwise hopeless cases. In case anybody is worried that the little baby, Louise, will develop some psychological problems upon finding out about her unique origins, Dr. Steptoe and Dr. Edwards have made it clear that by the time Louise is old enough to understand how she was conceived, there will be many more happy, healthy test-tube babies, and no one will think there is anything unusual about them.

The technique for making a baby in a test tube is called *in vitro* fertilization. *In vitro* is Latin for "in glass," and the term signifies that the events occur inside a test tube rather than inside the body. *In vitro* fertilization is merely allowing the normal processes of nature to take place inside a test tube rather than inside a woman's body.

Of course the baby did not, and could not, grow up in the test tube. It was merely fertilized, conceived, and then nourished for two days in the test tube until Mrs. Brown's body and uterus were properly prepared to receive it. Aside from those first two days of little Louise's life, she spent the usual nine months inside her mother's womb before the time of delivery.

At the same time that religious leaders, politicians, and just about anyone who was available to offer an opinion were debating the morality of a baby yet to be born, a New York jury was about to make a momentous decision that would influence the legality not of making test-tube babies but of interfering with the making of test-tube babies. A patient was suing a leading gynecologist for destroying the test-tube "embryo" which a member of his staff was going to reimplant in her uterus. She had been trying for ten years to have a child, but she had had no success because of hopelessly damaged tubes. It was not considered likely that her egg had actually been fertilized, but when she complained to the jury that this doctor "murdered my baby," it became a major test case in New York City.

Even though many doctors felt that the experiment on this patient did not have any chance of succeeding, and though the experiment did not have the sophisticated background of the work being done by Steptoe and Edwards in England, the New York jury gave a verdict in favor of the patient. This may indicate that no matter what politicians, theologians, and medical critics may think, test-tube fertilization is likely to become accepted by the public. The embryos conceived within test tubes are going to be considered living human beings, and though many of them may perish, people are more excited than shocked by the prospect of considering them normal human beings.

Why did one test-tube fertilization finally work successfully, and can it be repeated with regularity? Did Steptoe and Edwards just have one lucky case after years of failure, or was there a solid basis for their work, and did some modification result in the success with Leslie Brown?

Their experiments began a great many years ago and involved an incredibly complicated variety of techniques which had to be tested over and over again in animals before being tested in humans. Determining the composition of the fluid in which the sperm and egg are to be bathed, the best time to remove and reimplant the egg, and monitoring the hormone levels of the mother prior to the retrieval of the egg all required years of patient effort. As the doctors came to understand how fertilization takes place and how the fertilized egg implants in the uterus, they slowly simplified their techniques, and this greater simplification seems to be what was required.

The first steps of the process involve the doctor's inserting a laparoscope into the patient's abdomen through a tiny puncture. The patient is anesthetized, so she feels no pain. With the laparoscope the doctor is able to locate the follicle which is about to ovulate. With a tiny needle he suctions the egg out of the ovary, and transfers it into a dish which contains nutrients for both the egg and the sperm. In the meantime, the sperm have already been allowed to capacitate in their own dish for several hours. The sperm are then transferred into the dish that contains the egg. After fertilization, the egg is placed into another solution. The egg then divides into two cells, each of which then divides again—until after fifty hours the egg has become a little eight-cell embryo.

Two days after its conception this microscopic embryo, smaller than a period on this page, was placed in Mrs. Brown's uterus, and survived. Although the process of *in vitro* fertilization is complicated, each step of the way had been carefully mapped out over the previous twelve years. The simplification of the process is what finally led to its success.

The elegance and simplicity of the techniques for test-tube fertilization developed by Steptoe and Edwards do not require the bureaucracy of an enormous medical center. Research in this area will certainly be retarded in the United States, however, because in 1975 federal support for research into *in vitro* fertilization was halted because of a fear that such research was not ethical. However, with the success of Steptoe and Edwards and studies demonstrating the safety of this approach for mother and child, we may eventually see test-tube babies in the United States as well.

Now that we have already stepped over into that brave new world, think of the other possibilities. What if a woman has had a hysterectomy? She has no uterus at all, but does have normal ovaries and a fertile husband. It would now be possible to remove one of her eggs through the laparoscope, fertilize it in a culture dish with her husband's sperm, and then implant this new embryo into another woman, who could act as a "surrogate" mother. Then when the baby is delivered nine months later, it could be turned over to the mother who originally provided the egg. From the opposite point of view, what if a woman had a perfectly normal uterus and a fertile husband, but her ovaries were incapable of producing eggs? An egg could be extracted from a donor through the laparoscope, fertilized with her husband's sperm, and then implanted into her own uterus. The legal and social dilemmas created by such possibilities will probably not be resolved in the near future, but we do have the technical ability now to perform such feats.

## A Review of Fertilization

A human female possesses at birth her entire stock of eggs. These eggs have already completed the first stages of development prior to the woman's birth. During the woman's life, until menopause, these partly developed eggs merely await the moment of ovulation.

Early in each menstrual cycle, several of these undeveloped follicles begin to enlarge under the stimulation of FSH, the follicle-stimulating hormone released by the pituitary gland. Every month a thousand such eggs attempt early development, but only a few are able to form follicles, and generally only one is ovulated. The follicle is a bubblelike expansion of sticky fluid within which the egg is enclosed. It comes to the surface of the ovary just prior to the time of ovulation.

Ovulation is triggered by release of LH, luteinizing hormone, also secreted by the pituitary gland. The role of LH is not just to stimulate the release of the egg from its follicle (although that is the most dramatic aspect of ovulation). Just as important, LH stimulates the egg—quiescent for perhaps twenty years—to mature, and to reduce its chromosome number from forty-six to twenty-three. Half of the chromosomes are discarded, and the other half of the genetic material remains to await union with the genetic material of the sperm. It is only at this stage, after its maturation, that the egg can possibly be fertilized. Eggs that have not been matured cannot be fertilized in a test tube. There are elaborate methods for maturing immature eggs in a test tube and then fertilizing them with sperm, but thus far no such fertilized eggs from any animal have developed into babies. They merely mimic the early stages of fertilization, but never get any further. Thus the maturing of the egg under the stimulation of LH is critical.

After completion of maturation, the eggs are ready to be fertilized in the test tube. Watching the fertilization of an egg, the actual creation of a new life, is a startling experience. Once the sperm head reaches the interior of the egg, it begins to enlarge and swell. The membrane that surrounds the sperm joins the membrane surrounding the egg, and they seem to melt into one common membrane. The egg appears to swallow the sperm as the two separate cells become one. After the two cells are joined into one, the genes from the sperm and the genes from the egg enlarge and fuse together. Shortly thereafter, the cell begins to divide.

Over a period of several days, the two cells each divide, forming four cells; each of these then divides to create eight cells. The fourth division results in a sixteen-cell mass and the fifth division results in a thirty-two-cell mass, which is called the morula. By the time the next division of cells takes place, a small cavity forms in the ball of cells. This stage is called the early blastocyst. It does not resemble anything like a baby, but it is the beginning of life. Over the next nine months, different areas of this ball of cells will become specialized into arms, legs, a head, and all of the various organs. But at this blastocyst stage, when the baby is only about five days old, it is simply a ball of cells.

## Step-by-Step Details of How Human Test-Tube Babies Are Made

### ARE THE CHILDREN GOING TO BE NORMAL?

In 1974 Dr. Edwards wrote a detailed scientific article outlining why birth defects would not be a problem with test-tube fertilization. In fact, defective children might be even less common than with normally conceived children. In rabbits, mice, and rats, test-tube babies have thus far all been normal. Embryos of pigs, cattle, and sheep transferred to a surrogate mother also have developed without abnormalities. Embryos in their early stages are highly resistant to malformations, and although many of them fail to survive, the ones that do survive turn out normally.

### OBTAINING THE EGG AT THE RIGHT TIME

Eggs cannot be fertilized until they have adequately matured. The final maturation occurs just several hours prior to the expected moment of ovulation. To obtain eggs at exactly the right time, the doctor must monitor the changes in the woman's hormone levels. During the first two weeks of the woman's cycle, urinary estrogens are determined every day. When mid-cycle nears, and the estrogen level begins to rise, the woman is checked every three hours for urinary LH. The key to successful estimation of the time of ovulation is pinpointing the rise in LH.

Ovulation occurs rather predictably twenty-two hours after the beginning of the rise in LH. The eggs are therefore retrieved twenty hours after the LH surge. The egg is mature at this point and ready for fertilization.

## COLLECTION OF THE EGG

The long and slender instrument called a laparoscope is introduced into the woman's abdomen through her belly button, while she is anesthetized. The ovaries are examined for the presence of a ripe follicle. The follicle that contained the egg is thin-walled, blue-pink in color, and sits on the ovarian surface like a bubble. A small needle is introduced into the abdomen and carefully guided, using the laparoscope. The follicle is punctured with the needle, and the egg is removed by gentle and controlled suction. The egg thus collected will be normally matured and preovulatory. The patient wakes up very quickly after this operation and is generally ready to go home that evening.

The punctured follicle fills up with blood in a matter of minutes and turns yellow, forming the corpus luteum, which in the second half of the cycle will produce progesterone, the hormone necessary to sustain pregnancy. However, the progesterone production from the punctured follicle is often not as reliable as in the normal situation, and the woman is given supporting doses of either progesterone or HCG until the embryo has implanted.

## PREPARATION OF THE SPERM

Freshly ejaculated sperm cannot fertilize the egg until they have gone through a stage called capacitation. It used to be thought that capacitation could only occur within the female reproductive organs. Dr. Edwards, however, has demonstrated that in a simple fluid available in almost any laboratory (Tyrode's solution), sperm require just a few hours of incubation in the test tube to become capacitated, and thus capable of fertilizing the eggs. Since capacitation can occur so easily in an ordinary fluid, scientists now assume that there is nothing very specific about capacitation. Simply, a period of time is necessary for the sperm to shed a surface coat of inhibiting factors which would otherwise prevent egg penetration.

After the husband has provided his ejaculate to the doctor in a sterile laboratory jar, it is poured into a culture dish. The sperm are separated from the semen and rediluted to a concentration of about one million sperm per cc. Since in a test tube all of the obstacles normally encountered by the sperm in their transport to the egg have been removed, only a small fraction of the sperm are needed. Thus, test-tube fertilization may not only be a boon for women with hopelessly destroyed tubes, but perhaps also for men with very low sperm counts.

This all seems too elegantly simple. Prior to Dr. Edwards's experiments, when the popular theory was that capacitation of sperm could occur only inside the uterus, many vain attempts were made to fertilize human eggs with sperm taken from the woman's cervical mucus, or preincubated in an animal oviduct, placed in an intrauterine chamber, or incubated with slices of uterine or oviduct tissue. One of the reasons that Dr. Edwards was successful is that he was capable of simplifying the whole process of artificial fertilization, particularly sperm capacitation.

## FERTILIZATION IN THE TEST TUBE

The eggs, which have been collected approximately one to four hours prior to expected ovulation, are placed in a dish with spermatozoa that have been preincubated for two to three hours in order to "capacitate." Penetration of the sperm into the eggs begins approximately two to three hours later, and by twelve hours the first signs of fertilization and cleavage are noted. The whole spermatozoon, from the front battering ram, called the acrosome, to the tip of the tail, passes through the zona pellucida (the tough outer membrane of the egg) and ultimately into the egg. The egg is

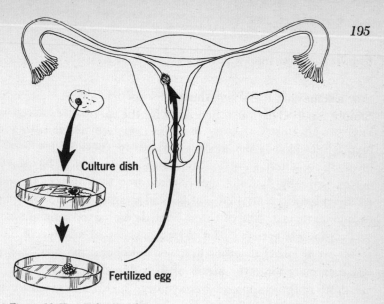

*Figure 18.* Test-Tube Fertilization and Implantation of the Embryo.

then transferred to a somewhat different solution which contains more nutrients, called Ham's F-10 solution. When the embryo has divided into eight cells, usually about fifty hours after the test-tube conception, it is placed into the uterus of the mother-to-be. Small supporting doses of HCG are usually used to make sure that the corpus luteum continues to make progesterone and that the uterine lining is maximally receptive to the ingrowth of the egg.

## PLACEMENT OF THE FERTILIZED EMBRYO
## INTO THE MOTHER'S UTERUS

The eight-cell embryo, having been checked carefully under the microscope to make sure all is well, is then transferred nonsurgically with a little culture medium into the woman's uterus through the cervix. Continued injections of HCG are given for the next two weeks in order to make sure that the uterus is properly lined by progesterone until the fetus is on its own. Two weeks after implantation, the embryo should be able to make its own HCG and therefore adequate amounts of progesterone to support its own pregnancy (Fig. 18).

## Test-Tube Offspring in Animals

There are two ways of producing test-tube babies. One is by test-tube fertilization, in which the egg of the female and sperm of the male are mixed together in a test tube, and the resulting embryo is placed into the mother's womb to continue its development. The other is by embryo transfer, in which fertilization occurs normally, but the embryo at three to five days of age is removed from the original mother and transferred into the womb of another female. The test-tube baby delivered in England in 1978 was of the first variety. The egg of the mother and sperm of the father were mixed together in a test tube, and the fertilized egg was then placed into the uterus of the original mother.

Both of these approaches have been highly successful for several years in animals. Science has actually progressed much further in this field than people realize. The reluctance to attempt producing test-tube babies in humans has caused us to lag well behind what has been routinely performed in animals for the past twenty years. It was known long before 1950 that simply by pricking a frog's egg we could make it develop as though it were fertilized by a sperm. Only the rare such egg ever developed into a mature adult frog, however, although many of them went successfully through the early stages of development and became free-swimming tadpoles.

Then in 1959 an amazing experiment was performed. Eggs were taken out of a mature female rabbit, mixed in a test tube with sperm from a male rabbit, and normal embryos developed through the first three days of life. These embryos were then transferred from the test tube into a different female rabbit's womb. The surrogate mother rabbit subsequently gave birth to healthy young. This experiment was especially dramatic because the egg and sperm came from black rabbits, and the embryos developed in the womb of a white rabbit. The white mother rabbit thus gave birth not to white rabbits, but to black ones.

One secret to the success of this experiment after previous failures was that the sperm were allowed to incubate for a period of time in a female rabbit's uterus. Thus the sperm were "capacitated" prior to being mixed in a test tube with rabbit eggs. Since that time scientists have learned how to capacitate sperm in a test tube as well, thus eliminating the need of running them through a female's reproductive tract. Bypassing the necessity for sperm to reside in the female in order to be able to fertilize an egg has made the concept of test-tube fertilization more practical. Test-tube fertilization is now an exciting, practical, and repeatable event in up to eleven animal species thus far studied.

Perhaps more successful than fertilization in the test tube has been the transfer of three-day-old embryos to the womb of other mothers. In 1962, fertilized sheep eggs from prize animals were placed in the fallopian tubes of rabbits and the rabbits were sent by air from England to South Africa. Once the rabbits arrived in South Africa, the prize sheep embryos were removed from their tubes and placed in the uterus of lower-quality sheep. This resulted in the birth of normal prize British Leicester lambs in South Africa by genetically inferior sheep that served as a "foster mothers." Cattle embryos, sheep embryos, and pig embryos are now routinely transferred long distances within the oviducts of rabbits. These embryos, usually from prize strains of farm animals in distant areas, are then placed in relatively inexpensive "breeder" animals that deliver prize babies when the pregnancy is over. Cattle and sheep embryos are capable of living and developing normally in the rabbit oviduct for three to five days, which is usually plenty of time for transfer over long distances. This is of course much easier than importing the sheep or the cows themselves for such breeding purposes. It also means that many more prize animals can be produced.

In 1976, prize horse embryos were transferred similarly in the oviduct of a rabbit all the way from Cambridge, England, to Krakow, Poland, a journey lasting thirty-three hours. Thus horse embryos, like sheep and cattle embryos, remain viable and develop normally for at least two to five days when stored in the oviducts of a rabbit during transport over long distances.

In all of these transfers, hormone injections were used in both the donors and the recipients to make certain they were at the same stage of their estrus cycle, and to ensure that the lining of the recipient's uterus would be at exactly the right stage of development to receive the embryo. If these two animals, donor and recipient, were not "synchronized," the transferred embryo could not successfully develop in the recipient.

For that reason, freezing of the embryos has become equally popular. Embryos can be frozen and stored for indefinite periods of time, thawed at a later date, implanted in a recipient uterus at any time in the future, and a normal baby can develop. In 1972 this technique was first used in mice. Over twenty-five hundred mouse embryos were frozen at the eight-cell stage and stored for eight days. After these frozen "babies" were thawed, a thousand of them appeared to be quite healthy, and were transferred into "foster mother" mice. Sixty-five percent of these foster mothers became pregnant with the frozen/thawed embryos, and gave birth to normal, full-term mice.

A protective agent, DMSO (dimethyl sulfoxide), was used to prevent damage that would otherwise occur from the freezing process. This agent was able to protect the eight-cell embryos, and the freezing literally held them in a suspended state of animation, waiting for the time when they would be thawed and transplanted into waiting mothers. In 1974, the same researcher again froze mouse embryos, but this time stored them for a full six months, and shipped them across the Atlantic Ocean from Maine to England, still frozen. In Cambridge, England, the mouse embryos were thawed upon arrival (189 days after the original freezing), and transferred into the uteruses of nonpregnant female mice. These mice then gave birth to normal young. This achievement was made even more dramatic by the fact that the embryos were from black mice and the foster mother was a white mouse. Since then sheep, cattle, and even rabbit embryos have been successfully frozen, stored, thawed, and implanted into nonpregnant females of the same species, with the development of full-term normal offspring.

Although test-tube fertilization followed by transfer of the embryo back into the mother has yielded low pregnancy rates, transfer of an early embryo from one mother into another mother yields extremely high pregnancy rates. Seventy-five percent of sheep and 90 percent of cattle so treated developed completely normal pregnancies to term. In pigs, the pregnancy rate with embryo transfer was close to 100 percent. The ability of fertilized eggs to survive in the oviduct of the rabbit for three to five days allows the transport of embryos over long distances with little cost. Though some of these techniques may seem a bit frightening, indeed almost like science fiction, they are being used every day with livestock. The application of some of these techniques to humans may solve infertility problems for couples who otherwise would have no hope.

But that is not where the possibilities end. There are unbelievable types of crossbreeding experiments presently being conducted. Generally the egg from an animal of one species can only be fertilized by sperm from an animal of the same species. For example, if rat eggs are surgically transferred into the oviducts of rabbits, who are then mated with male rabbits, the rabbit spermatozoa which travel the tube to find their way to these rat eggs will attach to the outer layers of the egg but never penetrate it. Only rat sperm would be capable of penetrating the rat eggs. However, some scientists have actually denuded the egg of its protecting outer layers (called the zona pellucida), and found that sperm from any species can then penetrate and fertilize the egg of any other species. In fact, recently a highly respected scientist has shown that human sperm can actually fertilize a denuded hamster egg. This experiment might terrify you into thinking some sort of monstrous hybrids could thus be formed by test-tube fertilization between species. However, none of these fertilized eggs has ever been able to develop beyond several cells, and no scientist seriously considers such a cross between species possible.

Yet there are some interesting examples of mating between different, but closely related, species. Certainly horses, cattle, sheep, pigs, dogs, cats, rats, and mice will not mate with each other, even artificially, to produce any hybrid offspring. However, the domestic bull can be crossed with the North American buffalo, to produce a hybrid called the "cattalo," which is a fertile animal that can breed further cattalos. A polar bear will readily mate with a brown bear, and lions will readily mate with tigers. In fact, when a lion mates with a tiger, the animal so produced, called a "liger," is indeed fertile and can reproduce more ligers. The elk of North America has been bred with the red deer of Europe to produce the "feral" of New Zealand. The feral has a voice that is a cross between the elk's bugle and the stag's roar. Rams seem to be successful in impregnating goats, but the resulting embryo invariably dies after the second month of pregnancy. The donkey and the horse have, perhaps, the most famous cross between species, but the resulting mule, though a viable and valuable animal, is sterile and unable to produce more mules. The zebra can mate with the horse and the donkey, so that one can have a "zebhorse," which is actually a zebra stallion that looks like a horse with stripes, or a "zebdonkey," which appears like a donkey with stripes. These animals are not fertile, however.

The major application of test-tube crossbreeding is to test more accurately the fertility of a man's sperm. If a man's sperm can fertilize a denuded hamster egg in a test tube, then he is very likely to be fertile. If his sperm are incapable of fertilizing denuded hamster eggs, however, it is probable that he is infertile even if he does have a lot of sperm.

## Cloning

Although most people still think of it as science fiction, cloning has actually occurred in lower animals and could possibly occur in humans very many years from now. Cloning is not like test-tube fertilization, which is essentially a normal conception which just happens to occur outside the mother's body. In test-tube fertilization the sperm from the male is mixed with the egg of the female in a test tube, and the fertilized egg is transferred to the woman's womb, where it grows into a normal baby. Cloning means that the egg develops on its own into a normal baby without being fertilized by the sperm. Cloning is an asexual, single-parent type of reproduction. There is no mixture of genes from a father and a mother.

The first animal experiments in cloning were performed in the early 1950s. Nuclei (the portion containing genes) of unfertilized frog eggs were removed and replaced with nuclei that were taken from the cells of developing frog embryos. Some of these frog eggs with their replaced nuclei, containing genetic material not from the original mother but from the donor embryo, acted as though they were fertilized, started to divide, and went on to develop into tadpoles. The frog is a particularly easy animal to perform this bizarre experiment on, because just by pricking a frog's egg, one can stimulate it to develop into a tadpole, and on occasion into a normal adult frog. Fertilization seems to be a mechanical event in frog eggs, and sometimes can lead to a completely normal baby without any contribution from male sperm. In another experiment, during the early 1960s, some biologists were able to take nuclei from intestinal cells of young tadpoles (not embryos), place them into unfertilized frog eggs, and again a few of these "cloned" tadpoles matured into normal adult frogs. Nuclei of *adult* frog cells, however, have thus far not been successfully used to "clone" unfertilized frog eggs. It appears that only the nuclei from embryos or very young frogs are successfully able to "clone" unfertilized frog eggs.

Eggs of mammals, or higher animals, are considerably more difficult to "clone." This is because frog eggs are about ten to twenty times larger than human eggs. Also, while tadpoles can grow into frogs easily in a pond or laboratory tank, human embryos have to develop inside the womb. Thus cloning in mammals or humans is a long way off. But scientists are getting closer. In the mouse, which is a much more complicated animal than the frog, and much closer to the human, eggs can be removed from a female shortly after they have been fertilized, and at this very early stage of development before the genetic material from the egg and the sperm have mixed, either the male or the female contribution of genes can be removed microsurgically. The cell then divides and the resulting embryo is placed into the uterus of a female mouse to develop. Using this technique, a few female mice have been produced by "cloning."

"Cloning" of a different sort occurs naturally in a few species.

The Amazon molly is an interesting species of fish in which there are no males. The female has intercourse with fish of a different species, and the sperm are not able to fertilize her egg in the normal fashion but merely stimulate her eggs to develop on their own into more adult female Amazon mollies. Because there is never a male contribution, there can be only female Amazon mollies, and they all develop by this sort of natural "cloning" method. This method of reproduction is more accurately called parthenogenesis. Unlike cloning, the offspring have only part of the genetic material of the mother, and are not an exact copy of her. In beehives, the queen bee and worker bees are produced by normal fertilization with sperm. However, the drones of the bee colony, the males, are produced by parthenogenesis, simply by the development of an unfertilized egg.

Stories about human cloning certainly make good cocktail party conversation, but such an achievement remains very far off in the future and may be extremely impractical even if the scientific problems are ever solved. Yet we do have a glimpse into a possible future when exact replicas of our cells could conceivably be created through great advances in the field of test-tube fertilization.

Test-tube fertilization, however, is real, and is with us now. During the next decade many women with totally destroyed tubes, or men with extremely low sperm counts not amenable to other treatment, may be able to have children normally, even though the first few days of their baby's life may have to be spent in a glass jar.

## Conclusions

In the last twenty-five years, scientists have been able to accomplish an almost undreamt-of miracle, the creation of life within a test tube. Although test-tube fertilization seems very simple, requiring just the mixing of sperm and eggs and the placement of the fertilized egg into the womb of the mother-to-be, the timing of these events is very difficult and important. If the timing is off, this seemingly simple laboratory exploit will not work. Most of the research that has led to the present success with this approach has been based on precise methods for obtaining eggs at exactly the right time of maturation, and replacing them after fertilization into the mother-to-be, again, at exactly the right time.

In farm animals, some astounding feats have been accomplished in the interest of improving the stock of cattle, horses, pigs, and sheep. Techniques for test-tube fertilization, transferring embryos from one mother to another, and indeed even to a mother of an entirely different species, are routine in the science of animal husbandry. What veterinary scientists have taken for granted over the last ten years makes our achievements in humans look meager. Some of the techniques developed in animals are finally now being used in humans, to alleviate otherwise untreatable cases of infertility.

If the wife has completely destroyed tubes, but she ovulates normally and her uterus is normal, eggs can be retrieved from her ovaries at the right time in the cycle, fertilized in a test tube with her husband's sperm, and several days later these eggs can be placed into her uterus via the cervix. Although there have been only few documented cases of such a procedure leading to successful pregnancy and normal birth, there are sure to be many more as the technique achieves wider use.

The techniques developed in animals could also benefit the woman who has no ovaries and no tubes at all, but a normal uterus. Her husband's sperm could be used to inseminate a donor female. The fertilized egg from the female donor could be retrieved about four days later from her uterus and placed in the uterus of the otherwise infertile wife. This approach is terribly dramatic, but it is scientifically possible and is done daily with farm animals.

A woman who had a hysterectomy at an early age but whose ovaries remained completely normal could also be helped. If she wished to bear children, it is conceivable that eggs could be obtained from her ovaries, fertilized in a test tube with her husband's sperm, and then the baby (who would have her and her husband's genes) could be transferred into the womb of a "surrogate" mother who would agree to carry the baby for nine months. Although this may never come about, it is scientifically possible.

Such approaches have been developed to a much more sophisticated level in livestock than in humans. With livestock, a prize cow can be inseminated with a prize bull's sperm, and the three-day-old embryo can then be transferred from the uterus of the prize cow to an ordinary breeding cow of little value. The following month, the prize cow can be mated again with a prize steer, and another prize embryo transferred to an ordinary breeding cow. These ordinary cows produce prize heifers, and the reproductive capacity of a prize cow is thus maximized.

Although most of these test-tube techniques are presently available only to a few, and although some may consider these techniques repulsive, they represent a technically advanced solution which may be the only help available to certain couples. Most of the scientists involved in this work do not consider it unethical if it provides a healthy, normal baby to a couple who would otherwise never be able to have one.

The political and ethical issues surrounding the creation of human test-tube babies have resulted in a complete freeze on government support of research on the subject in the United States, even though such research has been actively pursued in other countries around the world, and despite the fact that similar research on livestock animals is actively pursued in the United States. It would seem that if so much money can be spent on allowing a cow to conceive, perhaps it would be reasonable to expend as much effort helping human couples have babies. To enforce ignorance by restricting research is unfair to infertile couples; our only humane choice is to learn what wc can in these areas, to explain what is scientifically known and available, and to let couples choose for themselves whether to accept or reject such treatment. To deny patients an intelligent choice is to impose on them one's own metaphysical view of prenatal life, and to exclude them from the benefits of modern science.

# ·8·

# How Not to Get Pregnant: Birth Control and Sterilization

Recently, I was seeing a patient in the hospital who was about to have a varicocele operation in an effort to raise his sperm count. He and his wife had been trying unsuccessfully for three years to have a baby. The phone rang. He picked it up, and congratulated whoever it was that called him. After he hung up he gave me a disgusted glance and said, "Dammit, my best friend just had a baby." Not only did he and his wife have to suffer the agony of not having children, but they also had to tolerate the happiness of all their friends who had been having babies one by one over the last three years. Putting a chapter on birth control in a book like this may be agonizing in a similar way for some of my readers, and for that I apologize.

But the need for this chapter became very clear when an old friend recently paid me a visit. I hadn't seen him in twenty years. He and his wife had three children and wanted to know whether they should have a sterilization operation, or continue for a while on other methods of birth control. Ten years earlier they had been told by a leading authority on fertility that they would never be able to have children. My friend had had several sperm counts which he was told were low, and his wife had gone through every test imaginable, at a considerable amount of expense and discomfort. The doctor was rather gruff, unpleasant, and made her terribly nervous. Under the pressure of his unnerving bedside manner and the many poorly explained tests that she had to go through, her periods became even more erratic than they had been when they first went to see him about why she wasn't getting pregnant.

Despite much discomfort and many treatments costing a great deal of money, she still did not get pregnant. When they had their final conference with the "expert," he told them that her case was "hopeless," and they might as well just try to adopt because she would never be able to have children. She was furious. Yet the very next month, after giving up the thought of ever having a child, and in a way relaxing finally, she became pregnant. The next two children came in quick succession, and now, several years later, after being on the pill, and then the intrauterine device, with all the potential risks and side effects, she and her husband were considering sterilization.

The major problem of most couples in the world, even those who have had infertility problems in the past, is not how to get pregnant, but how *not* to get pregnant.

## The Male

### THE MALE "PILL"

Unfortunately, the availability of new kinds of contraceptives for men has lagged well behind those available for women. This discrepancy has been caused at least partially by an undeniable male chauvinism, but now more men are interested in assuming responsibility for birth control, as witnessed by the soaring popularity of vasectomy. Ironically one of the major reasons for the rapid early development of the female pill was heavy pressure and financial backing by proponents of the feminist movement, who felt that women should be allowed to control their own fertility, and have a baby only when they really wanted one. Now, twenty years later, men are equally interested in having a pill that can provide them safe, reliable, reversible birth control.

In fact it appears that we already have such a method available to men, but unfortunately it is in the form of a shot rather than a pill. In a careful study of twenty-one male volunteers, researchers have been able to reduce sperm production to zero by injections of testosterone every ten to twelve days. Less frequent injections, every two to three weeks, unfortunately allowed some sperm production to continue. Stopping the injections resulted in a resumption of sperm production and fertility three months later. Testosterone, the male equivalent of the "pill," is the same male hormone that is produced naturally by the testicles. The only reason that sperm production is curtailed by its administration is that it stops the pituitary gland from making FSH and LH, and therefore prevents the testicles from producing their own testosterone. The amount of testosterone in the body is perfectly normal, and the man's sex drive, libido, and sexual characteristics are unchanged, but the amount of testosterone present inside his testicles is dramatically reduced. All of his testosterone is coming from the shots rather than from his own testicles. Therefore, the man has no sperm in his ejaculate, but all of his male characteristics and his sexual ability are unaffected.

There are only two problems yet facing the widespread marketing of testosterone: it must be injected as a shot because it will not be absorbed from the stomach as a pill. Also, the large-scale studies necessary to prove its safety in huge populations are not being undertaken because of a medical-legal climate unreceptive to tampering with new drugs of any kind that might affect fertility. Yet injectable testosterone is widely available, and because of the great demand for male contraception, further clinical trials are an inevitability.

Merely reducing the sperm count to low levels is not adequate. The sperm count must be reduced to zero. When testosterone is injected every three weeks, the sperm count is diminished, but it does not go all the way down to zero. If testosterone is injected every two weeks, the sperm counts are reduced to very low levels (from one million to two million sperm per cc), which would make pregnancy very unlikely but still possible. When testosterone is given every ten to twelve days, the sperm count is reduced to zero and stays at zero as long as the drug is continued. On all of these injection schedules, the blood level of testosterone is no different than it had been before the men went on the contraceptive, and there are no significant side effects.

There are some oral "pill" forms of testosterone available, but they don't work very well. Halotestin is a chemically changed derivative of testosterone which is absorbed by the stomach but only lasts for several hours. A safe, normal dosage of this pill is totally ineffective in suppressing sperm counts. When the pill is given in four times the normal dosage, it may possibly suppress the sperm count, but it also results in liver damage. Remember that synthetic hormones carry side effects that the naturally occurring ones do not. So far none of the testosterone pills that have been developed by drug companies are very effective unless given in doses so large that they are toxic.

Of course, the female pill, containing estrogen and progestins, will suppress sperm production quite well, and would be as equally effective in the male for birth control as in the female. Yet using the female pill on the male would result in decreased libido and potency as well as enlargement of his breasts. However, some researchers are attempting to solve the problem by combining a very small dose of estrogen, much less than would normally be found in the female pill, with a safe dose of halotestin, hoping that the two drugs together would counteract the deficiencies of each one separately. The dosage of halotestin in itself would be totally inadequate to prevent sperm production but could counter the potentially feminizing effects of estrogen.

Any drug which seriously alters the amount of male hormones in the blood might result in decreased libido, and could also result in other behavioral changes. For example, male hormones tend to increase aggressive behavior. The elephant in rutting season is the worst example of this in the animal kingdom. He becomes an uncontrollable maniac, and would tear up everything in sight when his testosterone becomes elevated.

Another potential approach to the male pill is a drug, alpha-chlorohydrin, which has no effect at all on the testicles but which prevents the epididymis from maturing sperm properly. Theoretically this would be an ideal male contraceptive, since it would have no widespread hormonal effects but would merely prevent the sperm from developing the fertilizing capacity which they achieve during their twelve-day transit from the testicle to the vas deferens. Instead of a two- or three-month waiting period for achieving a zero sperm count, it would work in a matter of only ten to twelve days. The problem is that if the dosage is not regulated accurately, it can cause permanent blockage in the epididymis, which would be far more difficult than vasectomy to repair. Furthermore, in tests on monkeys this drug has caused toxicity of the bone marrow and a few deaths.

The most frustrating aspect of research on a pill for men is that there is already one available—but it is a shot rather than a pill. Though not formally approved by the government-regulating agencies as of yet, it appears to be a simple and reliable male contraceptive. When the effectiveness of testosterone as a contraceptive was first announced at the American Fertility Society meeting in 1976, one physician came up from the audience during the discussion and explained that he had voluntarily put himself on testosterone injections for the same purpose many years ago. He found it effective and safe. Since he was a physician, he could easily administer it to himself, and not have to worry about reprisals from the Food and Drug Administration. Thus a reliable and reversible male contraceptive seems to have been with us for many years. The only obstacles to its wide usage are converting it into a pill, which would be more pleasant, and performing the large-scale population studies necessary to make certain it is completely safe and achieve legal approval for its use.

## COITUS INTERRUPTUS AND CONDOMS

Coitus interruptus, or "pulling out early," is a dangerously ineffective method of contraception, since the portion of the ejaculate that contains the most sperm is that which comes out in the very beginning. Even the first few drops can often harbor much more sperm than the entire remaining portion of the ejaculate. Furthermore, sperm are able to penetrate the cervical mucus of the woman within several minutes. On a wide-scale population basis, this technique will reduce the birthrate, but it is inadequate for the individual who wants assurance.

Condoms were first used in the sixteenth century but did not become popular until the invention of vulcanized rubber in the nineteenth century. If condoms are used consistently and carefully, the pregnancy rate can be as low as 3 percent, but in actual practice the pregnancy rate runs closer to 15 percent. The heat of the moment, forgetfulness, and just poor technique make this an unreliable method of male contraception.

However, in Japan the condom (more commonly known as the rubber) has been spectacularly successful. In most countries the sheer inconvenience of the condom has been a deterrent to its use. But in Japan the condom's major disadvantage—its sheer clumsiness—has been converted into an attraction. A ritual has developed out of the use of the rubber that is much like a tea ceremony: getting it ready, putting it on, disposing of it, etc. Delaying penetration until the rubber is secured on the male organ has become, too, part of this mystique of sex, enhancing the total "experience," and thus adding to rather than detracting from the pleasure of the sexual act. The Japanese in this way seem to have solved a major family-planning problem that the rest of the world is still struggling with.

VASECTOMY

Vasectomy is the most popular method of birth control in the world today. It is a simple operation which can be completed in five to ten minutes in the doctor's office under local anesthesia with just a handful of surgical instruments. It is certainly one of the simplest and most common operations performed in the United States today. It requires fewer instruments and no greater skills than a dental extraction. Yet once the operation is completed and the patient's sperm count goes down to zero, he has greater protection from causing unwanted pregnancy than any other method of birth control would allow him. Furthermore, it requires no effort, no thought, and not the slightest inconvenience. There is only one problem: irreversibility.

In over half of the American couples who have been married more than ten years, one of the partners has been surgically sterilized. Sterilization in the female has become more popular in recent years because the techniques are simpler and less painful than a decade ago. Nonetheless, vasectomy still remains the simplest and safest of all methods of birth control. It is not usually adopted by couples who have been married for less then ten years simply because it has been considered irreversible. However, with new microsurgical techniques, vasectomies can now be successfully reversed in the majority of cases.

Unfortunately the vasectomy must still be considered permanent, because the vasectomy-reversal operation is very intricate and performed well by only a few surgeons. It takes only five minutes in the doctor's office to cut and seal the vas deferens. It takes two hours in a sophisticated operating room with an expensive microscope to accurately reconnect the vas. One percent of the men who desire permanent sterilization (and are firmly convinced they would never want to have more children) eventually change their minds. Thus a vasectomy, despite its supreme convenience as a method of birth control, and its improved reversibility, should not be taken lightly.

The vas deferens, which carries sperm from the testicles into the ejaculate during intercourse, is about one-eighth of an inch in outer diameter. Through the scrotum it feels like a hard copper wire. The inner canal which carries the sperm is no bigger than a pinpoint. It is easy for the doctor to feel the vas deferens in the scrotum and do the vasectomy through a tiny incision that hardly hurts at all. But trying to reconnect the tiny inner canal which carries the sperm is much more difficult and requires sophisticated microsurgery.

After vasectomy, the tiny amount of fluid that carries the

sperm from the testicles accumulates in the vas deferens. The pressure from this accumulation is not felt at all because the canal is very small. Yet pressure does build up and the sperm which otherwise would have gotten out stagnate and die of old age (the longevity of a sperm in the vas deferens is about two weeks to a month). The sperm then gradually decompose, much as our bodies do when we die. Fluid and sperm are reabsorbed to some extent by the epididymis, the canal that connects the testicle to the vas deferens.

Since only one-tenth of the fluid ejaculated comes from the testicles, the patient who has had a vasectomy notices no difference in his orgasm or in the volume of fluid in his ejaculation. It is simply all fluid and no sperm. A man notices no physical change in any aspect of sex, except that, because of the absence of sperm in his ejaculate, he is unable to impregnate a woman.

## The Female

### THE PILL

Birth control pills for women had their first clinical trial in 1958. Presently more than fifty million women throughout the world utilize "the pill" for contraception. When the pill first came out and was approved as safe, it heralded a new age in sexual freedom. All that a woman had to do was take the pill every day for twenty-one days of the month, refrain for seven days, have her period, and then begin again for twenty-one more days. The chance of an unwanted pregnancy was about one-tenth of 1 percent and there appeared to be no other serious risks (see Table 2). Twenty years later we all feel that we have been cheated a little bit. We came to expect easy birth control with no danger and no risk. We now discover that there are risks and side effects associated with long-term usage of the pill, but we have become completely hooked on convenient birth control. It has changed our way of life, and sparked a complete revision of sexual attitudes.

Most women will be on the pill for some period of time in their lives. Our society is addicted to a drug which is safe in the short run but poses serious long-term risks.

**Table 2. Rate of Pregnancy per Year**

| | |
|---|---|
| "The pill" | 0.1% |
| I.U.D. | 2.0% |
| Diaphragm with foam | 5.0% |
| Vaginal foam | 15.0% |
| Condom or diaphragm | 15.0% |
| "Rhythm" | 25.0% |
| Unprotected intercourse | 80.0% |

You will recall that there is no acceptable male "pill" at present because the active hormone testosterone is not absorbed from the stomach, and therefore has to be given as a shot. This was exactly the problem with the female pill until 1938, when the hormone ethinyl estradiol was synthesized. This is a very potent female hormone (estrogen) which because of a small change in the chemical structure is absorbed by the stomach. Another such estrogen, mestranol, was synthesized later. One of these two estrogen compounds is always present in any of the myriad different brands of female birth control pills on the market. Similar pill versions of the other female hormone, progesterone, were synthesized in 1954. Thus the major obstacle to the development of the female oral contraceptive had been overcome. All that remained after 1954 was to perform the appropriate clinical testing on a large group of patients.

Birth control pills represent a combination of synthetic estrogen and synthetic progesterone which suppresses the pituitary's secretion of gonadotropin, and thus prevents ovulation. Progesterone in the pill prevents the LH surge that would normally stimulate ovulation, and the estrogen component prevents the secretion of FSH, the hormone that would normally cause the ovary to prepare a follicle for ovulation. Estrogen alone, or progesterone alone, is not reliably effective, but the combination of the two hormones is. In addition to preventing ovulation, the progesterone component of the pill causes a thinning of the endometrial lining of the uterus, making it nonreceptive to implantation of the egg, and also produces a thick cervical mucus impervious to sperm penetration. Thus the estrogen and progesterone in the pill keep the uterine lining too thin for successful egg implantation, keep the cervical mucus too thick for sperm penetration, and in addition totally prevent ovulation by turning off the clock in the hypothalamus which ordinarily regulates the menstrual cycle.

Although the pill itself has some well-publicized risks and side effects, for most women it results in more comfortable and less heavy periods. Indeed, even for women who are not particularly seeking birth control, the pill is often prescribed for painful periods, heavy bleeding, and even acne. It is only long-term usage of the pill that carries much risk.

After the pill is discontinued a woman may not regain fertility right away. Eighty percent of women will resume normal menstruation and recover apparent fertility within three months of stopping the pill. Ninety-five to 98 percent are normal within one year. Approximately 0.7 to 0.8 percent of women do not menstruate normally after discontinuing the pill, and do not recover ovulation. However, this is probably less than the usual incidence of ovulatory problems in any population, and it is not clearly determinable whether the pill is responsible for these women's failure to ovulate. Fifty percent of women who stop the pill in an effort to get pregnant succeed within four months. After two years 15 percent of such women are still not pregnant yet. This correlates well with the known incidence of infertility in the population, and thus there appears to be no increase in the incidence or risk of infertility in women who have taken the pill. In any population, 15 percent of women who try to have children have great difficulty, and eventually need medical attention. For these women, fear of having an unwanted child is replaced by the fear of not being able to have a child when they do want one.

There have been many scares about side effects and potential risks of the pill, some of which are founded and others of which have no basis. There has been a fear, for example, that the pill may cause cancer. Since the pill has only been around for just over twenty years, no absolute conclusions can be drawn, but thus far there has not been any basis for believing that the pill causes cancer. Certainly in women who have breast cancer, any hormonal treatment has to be avoided, as it could stimulate its further growth. However, there are no good studies which demonstrate that the pill in itself increases the risk of developing cancer of the breast, uterus, or cervix. A number of studies have shown that there is a greater risk of blood clotting in the veins of women who are on the pill. However, the risk of blood clots in the vein is very small both in women who are on the pill and women who are not on the pill. It is just that the risk is greater in women who are on the pill. For example, 81 out of every 100,000 pill users per year will develop deep vein thrombosis, or blood clots in the veins. This is about five to six times the incidence of deep vein thrombosis in women who are not on the pill, but it still represents a very tiny risk. In fact the greatest risk to health in young women is simply getting pregnant. The risk of the pill must always be weighed against the risk of getting pregnant, which is far greater.

The use of the pill increases about threefold the risk of strokes in young women. These strokes occur in the blood vessels supplying the back of the brain, an area where strokes rarely occur in young women who are not on the pill. Although this is a rare complication, it is so serious that any woman on the pill who begins to develop difficulty with her eyesight, or severe headaches, should immediately discontinue it and see a doctor.

Heart attacks are five times more common in women over the age of forty who are still using the pill than in those not on the pill. In women who are over the age of forty, or have other risk factors such as overweight, smoking, high blood pressure, or diabetes, where the risk of heart attack is already somewhat increased, taking the pill increases it even more. There is even an increased risk of benign liver tumors in women who have taken the pill for more than five years. The pill can be responsible for high blood pressure in young women. The risk of high blood pressure is two and one-half times greater for women who use the pill for more than five years. Thus the pill has many potential side effects which are especially worrisome.

## THE I.U.D. (INTRAUTERINE DEVICE)

Even more convenient than the birth control pill is the device known as the I.U.D. (which used to be referred to as the "coil" because one of the first models was shaped like a spring). The first ones to become popular in this country were little plastic loops that could quite easily be inserted into the uterus by any physician while doing a routine pelvic exam. No one really knows why they work, although it was known even in ancient Egypt thousands of years ago that a foreign body in the uterus would effectively prevent conception. While early intrauterine devices were supremely convenient, they had a 2 percent pregnancy rate which, while fairly safe, was not nearly as reliable as the pill. Some women experienced bleeding, pain, and even spontaneous expulsion of the device from the uterus. Many women who had never had children before could not tolerate the device at all. Sometimes infection can occur with an I.U.D., and this carries a serious risk of scarring which could hinder the woman's fertility later.

Newer, much smaller I.U.D.s are now available that utilize either copper or hormones slowly released from the surface to help prevent pregnancy. Despite the improvement in these new models, the I.U.D. is still associated with a fair risk of menstrual discomfort, heavier than normal bleeding, and potential infection. Most women who have had one child and wish temporary but convenient birth control seem to prefer the I.U.D. to going back on the pill. They are willing to accept the slightly greater risk of pregnancy, as well as the risk of menstrual discomfort and infection, preferring these to the rare but potentially disastrous effects of the pill.

### THE DIAPHRAGM, FOAM, AND THE OVAL

Because of the risks of the pill and I.U.D., there has been a definite resurgence of interest in the old-fashioned "barrier" methods of birth control. The diaphragm and foam are well-known relics of a previous era and considered bothersome by many modern women. The risk of failure of either of these methods alone is about 15 percent per year, whereas when used together the risk of failure is only 5 percent per year. These approaches to birth control are inconvenient by modern standards, and can inhibit the spontaneity of sexual activity. Yet they have one gigantic advantage—they are virtually free of dangerous side effects. The diaphragm must be inserted over the woman's cervix prior to intercourse. To make it maximally effective, sperm-killing jelly or foam must be squirted into the vagina just prior to intercourse.

Recently a new development along similar but more convenient lines is the so-called "Oval," an oval-shaped tablet inserted into the vagina ten minutes prior to intercourse. The protective action lasts about two hours and is said to be more reliable than foam or diaphragm. The manufacturer originally claimed that the risk of pregnancy was only 1 percent per year, but some investigators have doubted that it is quite this good; although documented figures are not available, the Oval may well have a failure rate of 15 percent to 20 percent. Nonetheless the Oval, which destroys sperm upon contact and prevents their penetration of the cervical mucus, has no serious side effects and is more convenient than foam or the diaphragm. The Oval has become very popular in the United States and in Europe, where it is available as an over-the-counter item in any pharmacy.

RHYTHM

About the least effective birth control method is "rhythm." The concept behind this ancient method of birth control is that if intercourse does not take place during the most fertile mid-cycle period of the month, but is allowed to occur freely after ovulation, the woman's cervical mucus will be impenetrable to sperm invasion, and the ovulated egg will have become unfertilizable anyway. The second half of the monthly cycle, the luteal phase, is completely safe for intercourse. This method of birth control actually is moderately effective, and if properly done results in only a 25 percent pregnancy rate per year as compared to an 80 percent pregnancy rate per year when no contraception at all is used. Thus for large populations, rhythm effectively and carefully adhered to may result in a decreased birthrate. However, for the individual couple it is fraught with a high risk of pregnancy.

Rhythm birth control is exactly the opposite of timing intercourse to the most fertile day of the month. Using rhythm birth control, the woman takes her basal body temperatures not to try to have intercourse the day before ovulation, when pregnancy is most likely to occur; rather she needs to determine on what day her temperature rises so she can have intercourse thereafter when pregnancy is least likely. It is usually safe to have intercourse the first four or maybe five days after the menstrual period is over, and then to withhold intercourse until the temperature goes up, indicating that ovulation has taken place. However, if ovulation occurs a little bit earlier than expected, or if the temperature readings are not properly done, pregnancy may well result.

In animals, rhythm birth control would never work because the time when the female really wants to have sex is always just prior to ovulation, when she is most fertile. During other times of the month she will generally fight off any male interested in her. In a few animals like the rabbit, which seem to be ready for sex at almost any time, the act of intercourse actually induces the female to ovulate. Humans are strange animals in that we are the only ones that appear to have sex not just for the purpose of having a baby. That is why rhythm birth control can work with a moderate degree of success in humans but would be totally impossible to impose upon any other animal.

## TUBAL STERILIZATION

Just about the most popular method of birth control in the world today is sterilization. Its one disadvantage is that it has been traditionally considered irreversible. But for convenience, safety, and effectiveness, it cannot be rivaled. Just a decade ago sterilization in the female was accomplished through a relatively major operation requiring five to seven days in the hospital, a major anesthetic, and considerable pain and discomfort for up to a month afterward. With the methods for tubal sterilization now available, a woman need only spend a day or two at most in the hospital, and in some cases she may not even need overnight hospitalization at all. The pain is minimal and usually lasts only a day or two. Consequently, tubal sterilization is now even more popular than vasectomy as a method of permanent birth control.

The renewed popularity of tubal sterilization was brought about by the development of the laparoscope. Once the procedure is completed and the laparoscope is removed, the patient wakes up with very little pain at all. Previously, in order to get a good look at the tubes and to occlude them surgically, the doctor would have to make a fairly large incision. Now many patients return home within a few hours after waking up from the operation, and most of them return to their full normal activity within twenty-four hours. The incision is barely visible. This is the so-called "Band-Aid surgery."

Vasectomy is a safer and less expensive procedure because it can be done in a matter of minutes in the doctor's office without the patient's having to be anesthetized. Laparoscopic tubal sterilization still requires the services of a hospital operating room, and most patients will have to be asleep during the procedure. Still, this modern laparoscopic approach is so easy and so effective for the female partner that tubal sterilization is now slightly more popular than vasectomy.

Furthermore, if a minimal amount of tube is destroyed, the operation is indeed reversible in most cases with new microsurgical techniques. If more than half of the tube is destroyed, the success rate for reversing the sterilization is not very high. If only an inch or less of tube is destroyed, then the pregnancy rate after microsurgical reversal could be well over 80 percent.

Although most gynecologists performing laparoscopic tubal sterilization still use burning techniques which damage a large amount of tube, some may choose to use clips or plastic rings which damage only a tiny amount of tube. A woman who is about to undergo a tubal sterilization should ask her gynecologist exactly which technique he uses and make sure to tell him how she feels about it. For a young woman, particularly, it may be wise to have a less destructive sterilization procedure.

Tubal destruction may also be minimized by using a special type of electric current. The usual current is called monopolar. This means that it spreads outward along the walls of the tube from the tip of the electrode that grasps it. The spread of this current is a little difficult to control, and before the operator even has a chance to take his foot off the pedal that activates the current an extensive amount of tube may have been inadvertently destroyed. A newer type of current is called bipolar; this means that only the area of tissue right between the two electrodes is burned. There is no spread of current away from those two electrodes, and precise control is possible. Bipolar burning, clips, and plastic rings are all simple methods for accomplishing a "Band-Aid" sterilization without severely compromising the chances for later reversibility.

Perhaps more important even than subsequent reversibility is the fact that with the more controlled limitation of tubal damage, there is less likely to be inadvertent damage to other structures inside the abdomen. Although these complications are rare, it is possible for vital structures such as bowel, ureter, or even blood vessels to be inadvertently burned during a laparoscopic sterilization.

But not even sterilization is absolutely guaranteed. About two women out of every thousand who undergo sterilization will become pregnant. The tubes manage to rejoin each other almost miraculously. This is less likely to occur if the tube is occluded at its narrow portion, the isthmus. If it is occluded in the wider portion, then spontaneous reconnection of the tube is more of a possibility. It makes sense, therefore, to perform the sterilization in the isthmus.

Many physicians are now performing conventional sterilizations through such a tiny incision that the side effects are almost as minimal as with the more modern laparoscopic technique. This variation of the old conventional tubal ligation is called the mini-laparotomy. The mini-laparotomy consists of a small incision in the lower abdomen with an instrument placed through the vagina into the uterus which pushes the tubes up against the abdominal wall so that they are easy to grasp and divide through the tiniest possible incision. This technique works very well in thin women, but it is rendered almost impossible by the presence of layers of fat tissue. For this reason it has become exceedingly popular in developing countries, where the clamor for mass sterilization is sometimes great, where sophisticated instruments such as laparascopes are in short supply, and where the women tend to be thin.

ABORTION

Over a million abortions are performed in the United States yearly, and the number of abortions is increasing by about 16 percent each year. In fact, for every three live births delivered in American obstetric wards there is one abortion performed. Along with the proliferation of the pill, the I.U.D., and other methods of birth control, the legalization of abortion has contributed enormously to the shortage of babies for adoption.

Abortion is becoming a much safer procedure than it once

was. With the availability of proper medical facilities due to the legalization of abortion, the death rate has been very low and more women have come to regard the operation casually. Sixty-five percent of women obtaining abortions in this country are under twenty-five years of age. Seventy-five percent are unmarried and almost 70 percent have had no previous children. Women are continuing to seek abortions now at an earlier stage of pregnancy. Nearly half of all abortions in the last several years have been performed within the first eight weeks of pregnancy and 90 percent within the first twelve weeks.

The operation can be performed using local anesthesia or with the patient completely anesthetized. The most widely used method in this country is the suction curettage. The cervical opening is dilated with tapered steel instruments until it is wide enough to admit a suction apparatus, and most of the fetal contents are then sucked out. Once most of the contents of the womb are emptied, a sharper instrument called a curette is used to scrape the walls clean so that the patient does not bleed extensively.

Although a properly performed abortion usually does not lead to significant problems, there are definite risks even now that the operation is legal. As with any operation, there is a chance of infection, and any infection in the uterus can result in scarring of the uterus and tubes so that a woman can become completely sterile.

Certainly abortion has become one of the major factors in the control of our birthrate and population growth. It has been the bulwark of some of the most effective population-control programs in the world, such as those in Japan and China. However, it is, to say the least, an unpleasant event. It is unfortunate that it still takes precedence over less drastic but equally effective methods of birth control.

# INDEX

*Numbers in italics indicate the page location of illustrations.*